Hospital Ministry

HOSPITAL MINISTRY

THE ROLE OF
THE CHAPLAIN TODAY

◆ ◆ ◆

EDITED BY

Lawrence E. Holst

CROSSROAD • NEW YORK

1985
The Crossroad Publishing Company
370 Lexington Avenue, New York, N.Y. 10017

Printed in the United States of America

Library of Congress Cataloging in Publication Data
Main entry under title:

Hospital ministry.

 1. Church work with the sick.   2. Chaplains, Hospital.
I. Holst, Lawrence E.   [DNLM: 1. Hospital Departments.
2. Pastoral Care.   3. Religion and Medicine.   WX 187 H828]
BV4335.H673   1985   253   85-5688
ISBN 0-8245-0697-9

Contents

Foreword

Hospital chaplains care for others. Who cares for hospital chaplains? "Cares for" has a double meaning. First, it can mean "has an appreciation of." Almost any hospital patient who seeks attention to things of the spirit as part of healing has reason to appreciate the effective chaplain. "Cares for" can also mean "takes care of." Hospital patients rarely do that. Nor, for the most part, do religious denominations, governmental agencies, theological seminaries, medical schools, or other agencies which have some share in the world of the chaplains. Neglected by others, they usually have to care for themselves.

There are over five thousand chaplains in the United States today. It is hard to imagine these professionals not reading this book. In this very specialized field of hospital chaplaincy, they have not too much else to read. In recent years the sophistication of the Clinical Pastoral Education movement has helped fill the void on the library shelves. It has become a major morale-builder and "credentialling" agency, eager to generate standards in a previously ill-defined field. Yet Clinial Pastoral Education and hospital chaplaincy are not terms pointing to entities with identical boundaries; one cannot put an equal sign between the two terms to define them.

Before the middle of the twentieth century almost no literature on hospital chaplaincy existed. Curiosity led me to scan the field. In 1965 James Dittes and Robert J. Menges collated over seven hundred abstracts of research on *Psychological Studies of Clergymen* (New York: Nelson, 1965). They covered research on all aspects of ministerial work which touched on psychology, care, and cure. Clergy roles were part of the study. There were no index references to hospitals. Eighteen citations came under "clinical training," but only one of them was specific about hospital chaplaincy. Under the category of chaplain, or chaplaincy, there was a solitary reference. Much has happened, of course, since

1965, but the paucity of materials before that time suggests how little there is to satisfy the taste of historians or chaplains in search of their tradition.

If only the few thousand hospital chaplaincy professionals are interested in this book and it fails to find a larger market and readership, the publisher and authors will not be the only losers. Despite the sparseness of attention given the vocation, it is strategic. Its history and situation tell much about modernity and the effects of modernization on religion; about the ways religious people of vision have tried to bring wholeness and integration to life; about the difficulties of professional existence and the challenges to effective ministry and care.

To speak about the modern hospital chaplaincy is to locate chaplains in modern hospitals. Not often do most of us think how recent such hospitals are. In 1872 there were only 178 hospitals in the United States. In 1910 there were more than four thousand. This is a startling increase, and has little to do at all with the percentage of population growth in those decades, despite the great influx of immigrant groups to American shores. A revolution was occurring. Paul Starr in *The Social Transformation of American Medicine* (New York: Basic, 1982) has made a major contribution to accounting for that revolution. He pays due attention to the Catholic, Jewish, and a few other groups who built their own institutions to care for their own. Very rapidly almost all of them chose, or were forced, to take care of people outside their own immigrant-religious group. At that point, not having breathed a word about spiritual care of patients, Starr moves on to discuss the professional hospital concept.

When one thinks of the hospital through Western history and hears that religious groups were its main inventors, it is tempting to picture a somewhat more primitive version of today's hospital and project it back into history. Yet before the period between 1870 and 1910 or so, almost no counterparts to the modern hospital existed. Most hospitals were home-like almshouses, not scientific centers for technical work by physicians in highly administered situations. We cannot go looking for the chaplain, then, in the periods of Gregory the Great, the Protestant reformers, or the early evangelical and Catholic humanitarians, though all of them cared about care and cure.

When the modern hospital was put together, and as denominational impetus gave way to governmental, purely profit-making, or pluralist community motivations, the chaplain was rarely programmed in. We might compare the move to that made in the concurrent rise of modern universities. The old college, like the premodern clinic, was small and coherent. The new university, often under state auspices, was specialized and unintegrated. The hospital professions generated their own practices and ideology and these worked to exclude the religious professional. Of course, Catholic hospitals were operated by religious orders, and priests came to say mass or to share prayers. Of course, Protestant-based hospitals were in some ways extensions of the sponsoring churches' ministerial care. Of course, rabbis, priests, and ministers were ordinarily given clear access to patients from their flocks.

However, just as pluralist and state universities squeezed religion out of the classroom, pushed theology into satellite or alienated seminaries, and sequestered spiritual care in off-campus chapels, modern hospitals did not know what to do with the religious professional who embodied wholistic concepts of care. That is why the hospital chaplaincy movement, with its own professional norms and clarified ambitions, is not an historic form which got compromised in recent decades. Instead, it is a very modern, almost contemporary invention, still in search of itself. That is why a rare book like this which must necessarily draw on a range of talents, religious viewpoints, and specialties within chaplaincy, is so important. Some day individual theorists might be able to synthesize. For now, it is valuable to have these probes by numerous authors from a single staff, who give us the benefits of their interactions with each other, patients, and the hospital world. They are not capping a long tradition of buildings; they are still putting in place a foundation on recent footings.

What struck this historian as he read the collection of essays was the way they beckoned the reader into a world, a world at once familiar and arcane, graspable and intricate. When one drives past a hospital there is some awareness of its functions. Traffic jams at the end of patient visiting hours remind one of comings and goings by an outside world. The sirens of ambulances stir heart and soul to a tinge of panic: get out of the way for them, and hope you will not in any immediate future have to be in one. An illuminated cross might suggest a religious aspect, or the sight of a person in clerical collar getting out of an auto in the parking lot could underscore such hints. Yet the traffic lights change, one moves on and leaves that world behind.

When such a person becomes a patient, there is an entrance to a clinical world, one which demands the surrender of many stabilities that one takes for granted in the outside world. One may well have to yield clothing and possessions and carefully account for them upon return to the world around the hospital. Administrators turn one's identity into something on computerized charts. One gives up control of the daily schedule, is somehow at least partly rendered passive and submissive, subject to the technology and science of modern agents of care and cure. The passage over the threshold to the hospital world exacts a high price in terms of identity and tradition, zones where religion and spirit have much of their abode.

Inside the hospital, the chaplain in an articulated chaplaincy program is one of the rare professionals chartered to help the patient integrate the worlds within the hospital world, and the hospital world with the worlds from which one came and to which one hopes to return—to say nothing of transcendent worlds of meaning. Any set of essays that seeks to help define and refine the profession so strategically placed bids for the attention of patients, prospective patients, medical professionals of all sorts, and anyone who cares for the whole person.

The chaplain, as essays here point out, lives between various spheres of importance. Most religious professionals are defined by their congregations. Chaplains get their boundaries and expectations from the military, the university, or the hospital. That assigning of roles and missions cuts them off from others in ministry—yet not wholly so, for theirs is a ministry which must, in many senses, serve at least two masters: church and agency; in this case, hospital. Chaplains, therefore, also get their boundaries and expectations from "the church," the religious organization which regards itself as somehow related to the transcendent and where sanctions come through charisms, ordinations, vocations, and vows which are not always intelligible to the medical scientists or modern administrator. Yet this boundary situation signals the fact that in the world of patients, science and administration are not inclusive of everything.

I have spoken of the "world" of the hospital and of the chaplain. Familiar it may be, but neat it is not. In order to gain handles on it, one must bring to bear the many social, scientific, humanistic, and theological disciplines. In this book one finds reflected expertise in anthropology, sociology, and psychology. To make sense of the whole sphere, it is valuable to know some history, literature, and philosophy, for these and other humanistic disciplines try to evoke meanings which bear on hospitals and healing. Yet not all is theory; many chapters make it possible to locate this book under the "how to" category—not only "how to be a hospital chaplain," but how to be ministered to by one, or how to understand reasons for support and scrutiny of the profession.

So one will find here talk about chaplaincy and the anthropologist's cherished "rites of passage." This being a medically related text, there are case studies. Being religiously tied, it has to include some conversations about denomination and confession, though it is curious to see how much specificity drops, in the relation between chaplain and hospital and patient. Does the hospital threshold transform traditions and produce a religious world of meanings all its own, partly divorced from life in the congregations? If so, those distanced from the hospitals, but careful about religious meanings, have reasons to take notice.

These essays try to overcome not only specialization of the sort which forgets patients but also dualities which disrupt care and cure. Living and dying, mental and physical care, bodily and spiritual concerns, approaches to ethics and understandings, so often divorced from each other, intersect. Some of the essays are daring, for they show the chaplain pushing at the edges of the hospital covenant.

Some critics, typified by prophets like Ivan Illich, have scorned the whole modern hospital world. A number of essays in this collection suggest that, as expensive and apparently secure as it may seem to be, that world *is* threatened and its financing system and aura alike may be jeopardized. Prophetic criticsm of such an awesome institutional structure is constantly in order, especially from the sector of professionals within it, the chaplains.

Yet if anything of the free world survives and, with it, the ethos of technical and humane medical care, the hospital will not disappear; it will only be transformed. One hopes that in future transformations there will be more concern for the spirit and the whole human than there was in the earlier revolutions which produced the modern hospital. The chaplain already has a foot in the door of the hospital and is attempting to influence the impending transformation of that institution. This collection of essays bears out both their presence and their impact upon the hospital.

This book should hold interest not only for other professionals in the hospital, whose futures are intricately involved in this pending transformation, but also for the larger public, which has great interests at stake in the future of health care. The nature and quality of that care will be a vital national concern in the eighties.

MARTIN E. MARTY
The University of Chicago

Preface

This is a book about hospital chaplains—who they are, what they do, where they work. Despite their growth in numbers and their increasing professional competency, hospital chaplains, to many, remain an enigma. An enigma is anything (or anyone) that is perplexing, ambiguous, baffling, and seemingly inexplicable. In this context, it is the role and functions of chaplains that are enigmatic, not their personal characteristics. This book attempts to capture those unique, diverse, many-faceted functions. This book is intended for those who provide, receive, or in any way collaborate with the delivery of pastoral care. It is a book about the state of the art of hospital chaplaincy.

The chaplain's is "a ministry of dialogue." That is, it is a ministry of conversation, of the mutual exchange of ideas and feelings, both verbally and nonverbally. It is interaction around themes and issues that are determined to be important and appropriate by each participant. Dialogue, by its very spirit must be free, not compelled; mutual not unilateral. By its very nature, it requires both listening and speaking. Dialogue that is pastoral seeks to contribute toward another's personal awareness, understanding, growth, and integration in the emotional, spiritual, social, and interpersonal dimensions of life.

All professions in the hospital engage in dialogue with patients. But it is done in concert with other services and activities. Dialogue is the primary service and activity of chaplains. If not done with sensitivity and skill, it leaves the chaplain little else to offer. Further, if such dialogue is to be pastoral, its parameters must stretch beyond the patient's immediate illness and reactions. Such dialogue must be free to engage the deeper recesses of another's values and aspirations, hopes and disappointments, threats and meanings. In short, pastoral dialogue ought to give full reign to another's subjectivity. Whenever one is threatened and/or in conflict, one is suffering. To listen to the voices of suffering is the unique function of a hospital chaplain.

The purpose of this book is to explore and elaborate this ministry through dialogue. It seeks to do so by drawing upon the experiences and impressions of chaplains at a specific hospital, who—because of the size of that hospital's Division of Pastoral Care—have had the privilege of focusing their ministry upon specific and specialized clinical units.

This group of authors represents the diversity of the Division of Pastoral Care at Lutheran General Hospital. Two of them are lay persons, three of them are women. Denominationally they represent Lutherans, Catholics, Methodists, Baptists, Church of the Bretheren, Disciples of Christ, United Church of Christ, and the Church of the Nazarene. Such diversity of traditions breeds diversity of theology and practice. In addition to the twelve authors from the Division of Pastoral Care, four authors have other positions with this hospital: Carl Anderson (President of the Lutheran Center for Substance Abuse), Ray Carey (a research psychologist), Martin Marty (a church historian), and Ken Vaux (an ethicist). The latter two are consultants to the hospital's Project X, an attempt to study the interface of medicine and religious traditions. An elaboration of that project may be found in *Health/Medicine and the Faith Traditions: An Inquiry into Religion and Medicine*, ed. Martin E. Marty and Kenneth L. Vaux (Philadelphia: Fortress Press, 1982).

It is the hope of these authors that the reader recognizes those common human bonds that unite us all in our struggles with personal suffering and the vital contribution of religious faith to such struggles. To us that is more important than agreement with concepts enunciated in this book.

The book is divided into four sections. *Part I/ The Hospital Chaplain: Context and Identity* is introductory. It attempts to explore the dynamic, intersecting worlds of the hospital and the chaplain. *Part II/ The Hospital Chaplain: Listening to the Voices of Suffering* is an attempt to depict the unique and diverse expressions of pain. As one will see, those voices are as varied as are people.*Part III/ The Hospital Chaplain: Many Other Functions* seeks to capture the rich variety of a chaplain's ministry. Those functions are as diverse as chaplains themselves. *Part IV/ The Hospital Chaplain in the Future* undertakes the hazardous task of prognosticating the impact of the hospital's changing delivery patterns upon chaplaincy. Tomorrow's hospital will be the battleground where expanding technology will clash with constraining finances. Where that leaves the chaplain, and chaplaincy, is a crucial question that will demand thoughtfulness and courage.

Ten years ago a group of chaplains at Lutheran General Hospital attempted a similar endeavor. *Toward Creative Chaplaincy*, published in 1973, was the result. However, changing times and personnel, as well as new perspectives, have stimulated this new attempt.

Lutheran General Hospital has just completed its twenty-fifth year. In that quarter century our Division of Pastoral Care has received broad institutional support. Such continuous support has made our ministry and this book possible. Over those years much has changed and grown. In fact, those who return to visit hardly recognize our medical complex today. Two things have remained constant: suffering people still come to our hospital; our philosophy of human ecology* still motivates and directs our corporate energies. Because of such constancy, our Division of Pastoral Care has remained constant.

There are acknowledgments to be made: the hospital's board of trustees and administration, who have persistently supported an ecologic concept of care (that concept has provided the rationale for pastoral care); the staff (medical and nonmedical) and volunteers, who have accepted our full inclusion in the healing community (that support has provided the milieu for pastoral care); the patients, past and present, living and dead, who willingly trusted us with their most intimate concerns (that trust provided the mission for pastoral care).

To Dr. Wayne Oates, Professor of Psychiatry and Behavioral Sciences and Director of the Program in Ethics and Pastoral Counseling, University of Louisville School of Medicine, and to Dr. James Wind, Director for Research, Project X, Lutheran Institute for Human Ecology, Park Ridge, Illinois, who read the manuscripts and made helpful suggestions.

To my secretary, Fay DiNino, who not only typed manuscripts but whose own C.P.E. experience provided her a perspective and encouraged her "to make just a suggestion," many of which found their way into the book.

Not the least, to all members of the Division of Pastoral Care, past and present, student and full time, whose sensitive ministry helped "to write" this book, whether or not they are authors of a chapter.

LAWRENCE E. HOLST
Chairman, Division of Pastoral Care
Lutheran General Hospital
Park Ridge, Illinois

*Human ecology is the understanding and care of human beings as whole persons in light of their relationships to God, to themselves, their families, and the society in which they live.

·PART I·

THE HOSPITAL CHAPLAIN:
Context and Identity

1

A Ministry of Paradox in a Place of Paradox

LAWRENCE E. HOLST

A hospital is a place of paradox. A paradox is a statement or experience that appears to be contradictory, but in reality points to a larger, more comprehensive truth. A paradox holds together the seeming contradiction; it is the connecting link between the apparent opposites. To live is to experience paradox. It is to engage a world that is fraught with ambiguities, complications, and blurred realities. This is neither more nor less true of hospitals. Indeed, paradoxes are everywhere because apparent tensions and contradictions are everywhere. This year our nation expects to expend $305 billion (30 percent) of its total budget ($847.9 billion) on war machines. Why? In order to live in peace. Isn't that a paradox?

Alcoholics are advised that "victory" comes through "surrender"; psychiatry classifies some people as "passive aggressive," and as "manic-depressive." These terms suggest modes of behavior that are at opposite ends of a continuum. We are told that ambivalence (the tendency to harbor opposite feelings toward the same object at the same time) is all pervasive. We both love and hate those nearest and dearest to us. How is that for a paradox?

Paradox was not foreign to Jesus. Indeed, paradox was as familiar to him as was parable. He once declared that "he who finds his life will lose it, he who loses his life for my sake will find it" and, on another occasion, that "the meek shall inherit the earth." He promised to bring a peace that would surpass all understanding while also prophesizing that he would turn son against father and daughter against mother. By embracing such opposite views, he was pointing to a larger truth.

Portions of this chapter were delivered as the Russell M. Dicks Memorial Lecture at the annual convention of the College of Chaplains of the American Protestant Hospital Association, held in Kansas City on 27 March 1984.

We human beings are a paradox. We were created "living beings" out of dust and clay. It was a term used by the author of Genesis to describe all living creatures. Hence our kinship with nature. Like beasts of the field, we share common drives, protect territorial claims, are bounded by time, are given to die. Yet that doesn't fully describe us. We were fashioned in "the likeness of God." It was a term used in Genesis exclusively for human beings. The similarity to God is not a physical likeness, but a similarity of powers and capacities not shared to the same degree by other creatures. We are retrospective, introspective, and prospective. We are able to understand the processes of nature. We die like all living things but, unlike other creatures, we know that we will die. We are both self-aware and self-transcendent. We can both know and relate to our creator God.

So there we are, a created paradox: we have a kinship with creatures and Creator. We have divine aspirations and human limitations.

Though paradox is everywhere — within and around us — perhaps nowhere is it more personally and uniquely experienced than by patients in a hospital.

The Paradox of Crisis

To be a patient in a hospital is to be in crisis. The Greeks portrayed *krisis* as a paradox, containing a two-sided character: *danger* and *opportunity*. Indeed, crisis is just that. It is a fork in the road, a turning point, a confrontation that contains both *threats* and *possibilities*.

The threats of a crisis are apparent: equilibrium is upset; continuity is challenged; familiar routines are disturbed. Life can no longer be lived as it has been lived. Few emerge from a crisis unchanged, internally or externally.

This is also the opportunity of a crisis. New adaptations must be made; new coping resources must be acquired. That which has been destructured must now be restructured. The opportunities for revaluing, revising, reforming are countless; and many of the changes wrought in the heat of a crisis have staying power.

Crises are catalysts that draw to the surface the contradictions, the ambiguities, the paradoxes of life. They bring about a collision between our ceaseless cravings for control, stability, and permanence versus the realities of life on this planet that include chaos, disequilibrium, and upheaval. Whether recognized or not, crises are always religious experiences confronting us with what Charles Gerkin has termed "our infinite aspirations and our finite possibilities."[1] The encounter with human boundaries inevitably confronts us with questions of identity and destiny.

Crises confront us with still another paradox, namely, that personal growth comes largely through pain. One is not far into life before one discovers that the familiar and the secure must be relinquished in order to mature and to move on to the next stage of development. One had to give up the security of the crib to learn to walk. One had to surrender the safety of childish dependency to gain the autonomy of adolescence. In so doing, there were risks and pains, loneliness and confusion.

In *The Prophet* Gibran states, "Your pain is the breaking of the shell that enslaves your understanding."[2] He goes on to compare a crisis to a lobster. In order to fit into its shell as it grows bigger, the lobster goes through periodic shedding of the shell. During these times the lobster is vulnerable and in terrible danger. Yet in the inexorability of nature, the lobster must go through the crises of dangerous exposure or not grow.

Crises remind us of our paradoxical needs for both continuity and change. Without continuity nothing is rooted; our identity remains fluid. Without discontinuity (whether voluntary or not) life grows stale and dead. Like the lobster's shell, the old must be disturbed if anything new is to be evoked.

Crises expose the frailness and tentativeness of life. They remind us that nothing stays the same. In reality, life is no more fragile during a crisis; it only seems so because our illusions of invincibility have been swept away.

The Paradoxes of Hospitalization

In addition to exposing people to crises, the very context of the hospital poses other paradoxes.

A hospital is a place of life and of death. Most people in the United States begin life there (an average of 3,125,000 births occur in hospitals each year). Most people in the United States now die there (seventy-three percent of all deaths last year occurred in hospitals). We have tended to institutionalize both the beginning and the ending of life.

As numbers go, the average time an American spends in a hospital is infinitesimal. For most it is a mere parenthesis in a lifetime. It only seems long because the intensity of the experience is often far out of proportion to the number of days spent there. That, too, is a paradox.

The gamut of life, the beautiful and the ugly, seems to occur in hospitals. Life's contradictions are experienced there firsthand.

For some, hospitalization is a time of celebration: healthy babies are born; broken bones are mended; feared symptoms are diagnosed benign; pains are stilled. Hope abounds. God's goodness is apparent, or so it seems.

For others, hospitalization is a time of remorse: babies are born dead or deformed; feared symptoms are confirmed; breasts are amputated; injuries and scars are defined permanent. Hope is dashed. God is distant, or so it seems.

For some, hospitalization is a moment of preciseness. ("As we suspected, you have a hot gall bladder. I can schedule you for surgery tomorrow and you should be out of here by the end of the week.") For others, it is a time of disappointing impreciseness. ("We're just not sure what's causing all this. We're going to send you home and carefully monitor those symptoms. Right now we just don't know what else to do.") Some get answers they want; some get answers they do not want; others, no answers at all. The hospitalized patient also faces the paradox of being both free and bound. Never is one so free of life's daily demands as when one is in the hospital. All appointments and responsibilities are cancelled; sympathy, not obligations, is the order of the day. Yet never is one so bound as in illness. Schedules and services are devised by others. One's abilities and energies to attain certain goals, to experience certain pleasures and fulfillments, may be severely compromised. Hence, while being free of external responsibilities, the sick patient is internally constrained. In addition, the options for reengagement with life outside the hospital may remain highly tentative.

The hospitalized patient experiences the paradox of being alone within a myriad of contacts. One never lacks for company in a hospital. Indeed, privacy is rare. Yet in the midst of these human contacts, a hospitalized patient often ends up doing alone many of the things customarily done with intimate others, like eating, sleeping, watching TV, going to bed at night and waking up in the morning. There can be an eerie loneliness in the midst of all those human contacts.

At a deeper level, sickness often renders strange what has been familiar. Certainly, one inhabits the same body in illness as in health. But it doesn't seem the same. What over the years has been a trusted, predictable companion is now a stranger, emitting strange sensations and pain waves, causing shifting moods and a disconcerting drowsiness. In illness one is often not at home in one's own body. That, too, is a disturbing paradox.

In similar ways, one may not be at home with one's own feelings. The energy demands of illness often render one emotionally naked. Raw feelings of terror, guilt, rage, confusion surge to the surface in unprecedented intensity. Uncontrollable sobbing, torturous self-recriminations and dejecting apathy are not uncommon expressions of illness. Such powerful emotions can be unnerving and embarrassing, both to patient and loved ones. Nothing is under control—externally or internally—in sickness, or so it seems.

The hospitalized patient confronts yet another paradox that is more subtle and less easy to define. The vast technological resources made available to an individual patient are almost embarrassing. Rarely is life so highly valued. Yet, so often those vast energies and resources are devoted toward the disease of the person rather than toward the person with the disease.

Those of us who work in hospitals must confess that too often our medical technology prompts us to be more interested in kidneys than in the owners of kidneys, more preoccupied with the heart as a pump than with the heart as the seat of emotions.

This intense dedication toward disease, at the neglect of other dimensions of human suffering, is both flattering and disconcerting to the patient. It is, indeed, a paradox.

Eric Cassel makes a helpful distinction between disease and suffering. "Suffering," he writes, "is experienced by persons, not merely by bodies, and has its sources in the challenges that threaten the intactness of the person as a complex social and psychological entity."[3] As he notes, suffering may include physical pain, but is by no means limited to it. Suffering is anything that threatens the intactness and integrity of the person. It occurs when anything in which a person has made a significant emotional investment is threatened. It can, and usually does, occur on many dimensions simultaneously.

Hence, suffering, while universal, is deeply subjective and personal. It must be defined in a specific person, at a specific time. Personal meaning is a fundamental dimension of personhood and there can be no profound understanding of human suffering without taking those meanings into account.

The paradox in many hospitals is that disease is carefully, almost obsessively, monitored while personal suffering (as Cassel defines it) is largely ignored.

Finally, hospitals confront patients with the marvels and limits of science. That, too, is a paradox. Hospitals are society's extensions of its own "infinite aspirations and finite limitations." Many patients soon discover that a hospital's technologies are not infinite. And those limitations are translated into "medical failures." And those failures are absolute, for that patient, at that time. Little matter that a cure will eventually be found for that disease. What matters to that patient is that the cure is not available when it's needed.

Such is the hospital today—a place of paradox, of contradictions and blurred realities. A place where many of our patients' fondest hopes and prayers are miraculously answered. A place where many of their deepest fears and agonies are painfully endured. It is the place where hospital chaplains do ministry. And the paradoxes of that context cannot help but shape and define that ministry.

The Hospital Chaplain's Ministry

Who is the hospital chaplain? He or she could be from any religious tradition. In addition to theological training, ordination and ecclesiastical endorsement, that chaplain—in all likelihood—will have served a parish and experienced at least a year of clinical pastoral education, followed by certification by a national accreditation agency (i.e., the American Protestant Hospital Association or the Catholic Hospital Association). In most instances, the chaplain's authority will come from both the church and the hospital, though salary and day-to-day accountability will usually derive from the latter.

Though a member of the medical community, the chaplain's role is not primarily medical. The chaplain does not admit, diagnose, medicate, or discharge patients. What happens between the chaplain and patient will be determined by the needs, motivation, and availability of the patient and by the skills, sensitivity, and availability of the chaplain. Each is free to utilize or to ignore the other. No hospital is required by law or accreditation fiat to provide pastoral care. That provision is determined by individual hospitals, and its utilization is determined by individual staff members and patients of that hospital.

What does the hospital chaplain do? The answer to that question is the purpose of this book. The reader will discover that these functions will vary with individual chaplains and in response to various patient needs.

As a start, the chaplain meets patients at their level of immediate distress, seeking to comfort and sustain them. The chaplain will seek to engage the sufferer, to discern the patient's personal experience of suffering and to respond to it. If physical distress is seen as the precipitating event of disease, then suffering is the personal experience of that event. While both the physical distress and the resultant suffering are important, and intertwined, it is to the latter that the chaplain seeks to make a contribution.

As was previously stated, suffering has its source in anything which threatens the intactness and integrity of the individual. Since all dimensions of personhood are susceptible to damage and loss, so individual suffering has many potential sources and dimensions. That is the complexity and uniqueness of human beings. That is what makes suffering so deeply personal and what makes the chaplain's task so intriguing and demanding.

Suffering brings many things into sharper focus. It draws to fuller consciousness one's attitudes, emotional investments, meanings, and values. The intensity of suffering will be determined, in part, by what is being threatened by the disease; and what is being threatened by the disease will be determined, in part, by one's priorities; and one's priorities are determined, by and large, by one's values. So suffering, in its deepest sense, is a religious and moral issue, having to do with priorities, meanings, and values.

At this level, the chaplain best serves the sufferer by listening to "the voices of suffering."

What is being voiced by the sufferer through the suffering? What is the lament? The appeal? The anguish? The hope? These are most vital questions to the chaplain.

To listen carefully and attentively to those voices of suffering is the demanding challenge of the chaplain. And those voices will speak. The voices of suffering cannot for long be contained. Some voices will speak quietly and gently, others will cry out. Some voices will probe the mysteries, others will protest the injustice. Some voices will speak boldly, others tentatively. The tone and mood of the voice may be defiant or subdued, resigned or enraged, melancholic or courageous, angry or accepting, friendly or distrustful—or none of the above, or all of the above. The issue is not whether the voices of suffering will speak—they will—but whether those voices will be heard.

The very presence of the chaplain, and all the symbolic power it stimulates, will often provoke questions in the sufferer that have to do with origin and destiny, with existence and extinction:

"Something is happening to me that is causing me pain."

"Can I change what is happening?"

"If I can't change what is happening to me, who can? My physician, the medications, the chaplain?"

"If they cannot change what is happening to me, who can? Just who is in charge of what is happening to me?"

"If there is someone who is in charge of all this, why is that someone allowing this to happen to me?"

"Does that someone who is in control like me?"

"Is there anything I can do to influence that person in another direction?"

"What is my relationship to that power or force? What do I owe that person? What does that person owe me?"

"Does that person even care about me?"

The chaplain, as a living symbol of that living force, enters the struggle, hears the cries, discerns the questions, listens to the story. Within the limits of one's humanity, the chaplain joins the person in that pilgrimage of mystery and paradox. That pilgrimage did not begin in the hospital; it was only sharpened and intensified there. For it is not life and health, but vital anguish that gives rise to such awareness. Confronted by the threats of radical dependence and disintegration, surrounded by potential losses and dangers, compelled to acknowledge human boundaries and vulnerabilities, the suffering person cries out for deliverance.

The struggle is intense and personal. When one enters the privacy of another's suffering, one is indeed on sacred ground. It is to suffering that one's deepest fears and profoundest hopes are inextricably bound. To engage that struggle is to engage persons at the core of their existence.

In this struggle the questions exceed the answers, the mysteries enshroud understanding. This often wearies the sufferer and frustrates the chaplain. How tempting it is to short-circuit the agonizing pilgrimage with easy answers, to divert the sufferer's profound quest with shallow reassurances.

Yet, the chaplain is not there to remove suffering so much as to help people find its deeper meaning for their lives. This is done, in part, by reassuring the sufferer that the struggle is worth it, that meaning is ultimately to be found because God has deemed the sufferer to be meaningful.

Through one's personal presence, and all that symbolizes, the chaplain seeks to make God's redemptive love more real to the sufferer. The chaplain brings a simple but powerful word: "Yahweh's mercy is not an end. It is new every morning, therefore there is hope" (Lam 3:22-24). Indeed, such powerful words do not banish the mysteries and paradoxes — the finite boundaries and vulnerabilities remain — but they better enable one to endure and to persevere and to respond with integrity and hope.

So in a real sense, the paradoxes confronted within a hospital are the paradoxes of life: suffering people's infinite aspirations running smack up against their finite boundaries. It's as simple and as complex as that. It's an ageless struggle, true for all peoples, for all generations, and no less true for us — in or out of the hospital.

Hospitals do not create paradoxes and mysteries; they merely focus them. Suffering dispels the illusion that we are infinite, without limits. In that regard, suffering can be a great moment of truth for the sufferer. It is the hospital chaplain's privilege and responsibility to share in that rich moment of truth.

NOTES

1. Charles V. Gerkin, *Crisis Experience in Modern Life: Theory and Theology for Pastoral Care* (Nashville: Abingdon, 1979), p. 20.

2. Kahlil Gibran, *The Prophet* (New York: Alfred A. Knopf, 1923), p. 52.

3. Eric Cassel, "The Nature of Suffering and the Goals of Medicine," *New England Journal of Medicine* 306, no. 11 (March 1983): 639.

2
The Hospital Chaplain: Between Worlds

LAWRENCE E. HOLST

If the hospital is a place of paradox for its patients, it is not less so for its chaplains. However, the paradox is experienced in somewhat different ways. That paradox or tension is most dynamically experienced in the dual identity of the chaplain. The hospital chaplain walks between two worlds: religion and medicine. To put it in more political language, between two monolithic structures: the church and the hospital.

Each world, or structure, has its own domain and demands, its assumptions and mission. Each needs the support of, but independence from, the other. Often these worlds are complementary; sometimes they are in conflict. Always their interaction requires careful exploration.

The chaplain has allegiance to both worlds and both worlds have an allegiance to the chaplain. By training, history, and ordination, the chaplain feels a deep kinship to the church; but the chaplain's daily interactions are in the hospital, as well as are the chaplain's accountability to and salary from the hospital.

To move between these two worlds that are so markedly different — yet were at one time united — is to be in tension. The tension can be painful, confusing, exciting, creative. Like many tensions, it is never fully resolved and perhaps never will or should be.

The tensions that the chaplain experiences in walking between these two worlds can be identified in four categories: (1) the context of the hospital; (2) the chaplain's specialized training; (3) the strong influence of psychology in the chaplain's ministry; (4) medicine's and religion's conflicting perspectives.

Portions of this chapter appeared in *Health/Medicine and the Faith Traditions: An Inquiry into Religion and Medicine*, ed. Martin E. Marty and Kenneth L. Vaux (Philadelphia: Fortress Press, 1982), and is used with permission of the Lutheran Institute of Human Ecology, Inc.

The Context of the Hospital Fosters In-Betweenness

Most hospital chaplains began their ministry somewhere in a parish. It was a setting where they had primacy and where most of their pastoral care was rendered to people of a similar faith who held membership in a single congregation. They can well recall that a formal installation service on a Sunday morning suddenly provided them with pastoral authority and responsibility. A covenant was established; mutual claims were affirmed.

The hospital chaplain can also recall from that parish ministry spending much time in groups (e.g., public worship, Bible classes, boards and committees). Ministry to individual parishioners (in or outside the hospital), was supported by the formal structures of worship and usually included elements from those structures like prayer, Scripture reading, confession-absolution, the administration of the sacraments. It was a natural transition from the formal setting of congregational worship to the informal setting of individual pastoral care. Pastor and parishioner then shared as a dyad what both had shared many times as members of a worshiping community.

Recalling those days in the parish, the hospital chaplain remembers how gracefully ministry was accepted, how minimal was the role confusion.

In the hospital the chaplain is in a different context. Instead of chancels and pulpits, one is at bedsides, in recovery and emergency rooms, spending more time reading patient charts than the Scriptures. It is a world in which the chaplain feels little primacy. Certainly, in this setting the chaplain is not treated with the reverence and favor to which one had grown accustomed in the parish. It is a much lonelier world, one without the mutual covenants and support of a worshiping community. In a setting where tasks are so carefully delineated and precisely measured, the chaplain feels out of place.

No longer is role assumed. It is questioned and challenged. "What are you going to do for my patient, chaplain?" is not an uncommon question.

Nor does the chaplain have unilateral access to the patient. That access is shared with many: physicians, nurses, social workers, nutritionists, physical-occupation-speech therapists. Who does what to whom, and when, needs to be defined — and scheduled. Gone, too, is the homogeneity of membership in a single parish. The chaplain's "congregation" comes from a variety of backgrounds, representing a broad spectrum of faiths, or no faith. In a sense, the hospital chaplain is nobody's pastor and everybody's pastor. Gone, too, is the familiarity of a prior relationship with parishioners. Gone, too, is the authority bequeathed through installation. The chaplain has no claim upon the patient and can assume no authority, except perhaps a symbolic one. Patients come to hospitals for medical care not pastoral care. It is the physician they have "installed" and imbued with authority. It is to the physician that the patient raises those most immediate and urgent questions: "What is wrong with me?" "Will it hurt?" "Will I get better?"

Though a member of the medical community, the chaplain's role is not medical. Rarely is the chaplain seen as a decisive factor in such initial, crucial issues as diagnosis, tests, treatment plans, length of hospitalization, prognosis, pain control, diet, medications, costs, discharge.

Nor can the hospital chaplain even presume a religious motivation within patients. In fact, if one serves a large metropolitan hospital one will learn that under 50 percent of the patients identify church membership in their admission procedure. Accordingly, the chaplain cannot assume that traditional faith resources and religious rituals will be welcome or meaningful to all patients. This means that much time must be spent getting acquainted and developing "a feel" for the religious needs and meanings of each patient.

This takes time, and the chaplain quickly discovers that time is crucial in hospital ministry. Hospitalizations average seven to nine days (and are going down). Indeed, at best, the chaplain's is "a parenthesis ministry." Yet during that week in a person's life, the chaplain has the rare opportunity to focus considerable energies upon that relationship. Just as the chaplain is spared the myriad of organizational-administrative responsibilities of the parish pastor, so he or she is spared the technical demands of medical management within the hospital. In a setting highly endowed with expensive and elaborate equipment, the chaplain uses none. More often than not, the chaplain enters the patient's room empty-handed. Nor is the chaplain expected to inject, extract, to weigh, count, or measure anything. Accrediting agencies, state regulatory bodies, federal laws do not require that a chaplain make entries on a chart, much less even be present in the hospital. No hospital forfeits third-party reimbursement by failing to provide pastoral care.

Hence, the hospital chaplain is one of the few people in the pressurized, urgent, regimented clinical world of a hospital who may wander its corridors, move in and out of patients' rooms (invited or not), pull up a chair, and "just" visit. For the hospital chaplain conversation with the patient is not incidental to the completion of some other task; it is the task. And the chaplain has the time and freedom to devote to that task.

Though limited to the parenthesis of hospitalization, this confinement actually offers some advantages to the chaplain. In such time-limited encounters there is no "debris" from prior contacts, no obligations for the future. The chaplain-patient encounter can be focused upon the present. Past images do not need to be maintained. Threats of future recriminations do not need to be feared. This is important because illness unmasks people, frequently exposing raw, primitive emotions. In the relative anonymity of a chaplain-patient relationship these can be unashamedly expressed. The possibilities for candor are rich; the potential for posthospital embarrassment is minimal. The two of them (chaplain and patient) are not likely to meet again.

Of course it is not all so simple. The context of anonymity alone is not sufficient to guarantee openness. Openness requires sensitive listening, accurate empathy, nonpossessive warmth on the part of the chaplain, and the capacity for trust and risk on the part of the patient.

In a sense, the chaplain walks in that critical interim in a patient's life between a preillness state for which the patient yearns and a posthospital state which the patient fears. That interim provides the patient's first exposure after "the assault" upon the body: the malignant tumor, the coronary, the hysterectomy, the colitis, the mastectomy, the colostomy. It can be a distinctive time — a time when appearances are altered and plans are revised.

Such is the ministry of the hospital chaplain, extemporaneous, informal, casual, conversational. It does seem out of character for a hospital, doesn't it? Little wonder that the chaplain is often an enigma to the hospital. Medical personnel may and do question the chaplain's relevance. Yet, it is doubtful that it can or should be any other way. For while the chaplain is *in* the hospital, the chaplain is not *of* the hospital. At best the chaplain is between the hospital and the church. For that reason, the chaplain will always be somewhat in tension with the assumptions, values, and perspectives of the hospital.

The Chaplain's Specialized Training Fosters In-Betweenness

Prior to the 1940s there was no formal training for institutional chaplaincy. Two factors changed this: the advent of a clinical training process for clergy in 1925; and the development of organizations to certify hospital chaplains on the basis of such training in the 1950s.

Like the parish pastor, the hospital chaplain's preparation for ministry occurred in a seminary, with a major emphasis upon biblical theology, dogmatics, church history, philosophy, the arts and humanities. The educational process was didactic, cognitive, and deductive. But preparation for chaplaincy occurred in a hospital, with a major emphasis upon psychology, psychodynamics, and psychopathology. That educational process was inductive, experiential, and clinical. Each preparation was vital, though different.

The educational process most responsible for the training of hospital chaplains has been Clinical Pastoral Education, which began in 1925 in a state mental hospital in Worcester, Massachusetts. In part, it grew out of dissatisfaction with traditional theological education of the day, considered by many to be too abstract, too removed from life, too divorced from the practical tasks of ministry. Clinical Pastoral Education (C.P.E.) was an effort to get theological students out of their classrooms and chapels into the wards and clinics that house suffering people. As one of its founders, Anton Boisen, a Congregational minister, said on the occasion of that movement's twenty-fifth anniversary in 1950:

> This movement has no new gospel to proclaim, we are not seeking to introduce anything into the theological curriculum beyond a new approach to some ancient problems. We are trying, rather, to call attention back to the central task of the Church, that of saving souls, and to the central problem of theology, that of sin and salvation. What is new is the attempt to begin with the study of the living human documents rather than with books and to focus attention upon those who are grappling desperately with the issues of spiritual life and death.

In some ways that statement by Boisen was conservative—he was not introducing new subjects. But in another respect it was radical—it proposed a clinical method of learning that challenged the basic structures of theological education.

Boisen and others in the C.P.E. movement attempted to stimulate pastors to explore their own inner world in order to become more sensitive companions to others' struggles with the vital issues of life. C.P.E. boldly attempted to link the external and internal world of the learner, the cognitive with the emotive, theory with practice, theology with psychology. At least four major intellectual streams provided the context and impetus for C.P.E. in the 1920s and 1930s:

Theological liberalism saw itself as a reaction against the authoritarianism, the sterile dogmatism of religion. Optimistic in its view of human nature, social in its outlook, liberalism focused upon the internal authority of one's personal religious experience, rather than upon the external authority of church dogma.

Philosophic pragmatism espoused a scientific, empirical method of learning that focused more upon function than theory. Its approach was clinical and inductive; its goal was to increase functional competency.

It was an era of professionalism. The American Bar Association was organized, the American Medical Association was being reorganized, and an accreditation agency for public school teachers was being formed. In addition, the professions of social work and public health were taking root and being accredited. The pastor, once the most learned person in the community, was now perceived as professionally inferior to these other established and newly founded professions.

Psychology included many schools and emphases. Most of them inferred that in all of us there is an unconscious which houses the dark, irrational drives, passions, and impulses that are pressing for expression. It was a grim challenge to a world that assumed behavior was totally under conscious, rational control.

Less optimistic about human nature than theological liberalism, most of these psychological schools called for a careful study and analysis of the individual, particularly of one's competing-conflicting intrapsychic forces. Freudian psychology, in particular, introduced us to a rich new vocabulary: id, superego, repression, displacement, libido, cathexis, transference, defense mechanisms.

Religious existentialism, like many schools of psychology, was individual in its orientation and, like theological liberalism, was antiauthoritarian. It blended optimism and pessimism; it viewed human beings as free and responsible to make life's decisions, but without adherence to objective standards and without certainty of the outcome of such decisions. Humans were seen as both self-authenticating and lonely. Likewise, existentialism — somewhat akin to theological liberalism — placed more emphasis upon the human religious experience than upon the nature of God.

From each of these philosophic movements, C.P.E. borrowed certain emphases: from *theological liberalism* came the emphasis upon individual experience; from *philosophic pragmatism* came the emphasis upon the empirical-clinical learning method; from *psychology* came the emphasis upon the inner dynamic world; from *religious existentialism* came the emphasis upon individual freedom and the responsibility to authenticate one's own decisions.

No doubt the borrowing was selective, and no doubt there were other forces and influences. How and why C.P.E. developed as it did is a matter of conjecture. That it has profoundly impacted theological education and hospital chaplaincy is beyond debate. By participating in this process — and experiencing its double impact upon education and pastoral care — hospital chaplains again find themselves "in-between."

The Influence of Psychology Fosters In-Betweenness

An ongoing criticism of hospital chaplaincy has been its seemingly uncritical embracement of psychology. Rather than informing theology, many feel psychology has *become* the chaplain's theology. Whether or not one agrees with the indictment, it is understandable how such a strong influence occurred. Not feeling fully equipped for ministry in the clinical world, the chaplain turned to the clinical world for help. Psychology became a vital part of the chaplain's preparation and has provided skills that were needed, readily discernible and marketable in the clinical setting. Psychology has provided fresh insights into human dilemmas. While theology has historically portrayed the human race in a state of sinful rebellion, psychology has pictured the chaos graphically: humanity enmeshed in a biological order that includes primitive, conflicting forces not always within conscious control, struggling to gratify instincts within the prohibitions of society while making the necessary displacements of psychic energy.

Without doubt, psychology has deepened the chaplain's understanding of such internal psychodynamics. Unlike theological language, which tended to isolate the chaplain, psychological language provided a vocabulary that could be readily shared with other clinicians. As a result, the chaplain came to feel affiliation with a clinical team — sharing a common language and skills.

In addition, however, the chaplain was challenged to examine critically many of the church's traditional means and methods of ministry. Or, to put it somewhat differently, insights from the field of psychology have put the chaplain in tension with some traditional pastoral role models.

One such insight is the effect upon personal faith of psychology's understanding of personality development. While viewing faith as a gift of the Holy Spirit, the church has traditionally focused more upon the *content* of faith than upon how one develops the aptitude or disposition for faith. Since faith and beliefs were perceived to be identical and closely tied to doctrinal formulations, the church has assumed that faith can be taught. Such an assumption presumed that knowledge leads to assent and assent leads to trust; an act of the intellect is followed by an act of the will, which is followed by trust.[1] As Thomas Droegge notes, such a sequence does pose problems for a tradition that practices infant baptism, since such a practice suggests a reversal of order: trust preceding knowledge or assent.

But how does one develop trust? To this question psychology has much to say. In what one trusts—that is, the source and object of trust—is a religious issue; but how one grows to be a trusting person is very much a psychological function. Psychology has helped us to see that trust is not innate, rather it is "learned" by and through experience; and that such experiences begin very early in the developmental processes of the individual.

What is being suggested here is that historically the church has tended to place more emphasis upon the source, content, and object of trust (or faith) than in the psychological processes that help one to become a trusting person.

The influence of psychology in a chaplain's training has brought some "correctives" to that emphasis upon the *content* of faith. There are, however, dangers to any corrective. A chaplain, strongly influenced by psychology, might be more likely to see the church's tendency to separate faith from personality development, than to sense a tendency to "overpsychologize" religious faith.

Psychology helps us to see the human forces in the development of trust. We know how trust comes. It comes essentially through human relationships, especially early ones. Long before a child can speak or conceptualize, the child has experienced the whole gamut of emotions: love-hate, acceptance-rejection, trust-mistrust, order-chaos, pleasure-pain, reward-punishment. This means that long before the child can identify the experience, it has already been experienced.

We know what breeds trust: availability of emotionally generous, loving, caring, trustworthy people who are able to communicate these qualities nonverbally and experientially to the child.

We also know that not every experience evokes trust. There are times in every child's life when one feels abandoned, mistreated, unprotected and totally vulnerable. When the fund of basic mistrust is greater than the supply of basic trust, a feeling of insecurity and estrangement can result.

How fixed these early developmental patterns become, and how much room there is for later modification, is a matter of debate. That the early stages of development are important to the development of personality and character structure is, I think, indisputable.

What does all this have to do with pastoral care? A great deal. Certainly, pastoral practice has been influenced by these psychological insights. Certainly, they have caused many to challenge some of the church's traditional means and methods of ministry. In particular, many, in and out of specialized ministries, have come to question the church's heavy reliance upon kerygma (verbal proclamation). There are those who feel that kerygma must be a vital part of every act of pastoral care. Whereas chaplains, influenced by psychology, tend to feel that any pastoral act needs to be sensitive to the internal dynamics of the recipients.

When greater focus is given to those internal dynamics, then it becomes more apparent that the message (kerygma) sent by the church is not always the message received. This is not due to any deficiency in the message, and not necessarily due to any fault in the message sender (the proclaimer). Rather, it has more to do with the internal predisposition and dynamics of the receiver.

Words are symbols. What they symbolize to the hearer is determined not only by the message or the intent of the sender, but by the perceptions, associations, and past experiences of the receiver. Accordingly, words identify but do not necessarily create an experience. The words *God loves you* do not create love. Rather, they identify the nature of a relationship. If love has been experienced, these words are more likely to take on the meaning intended. The point is: how each person has experienced love at a human level will in all likelihood provide the context for grasping those words which describe divine love.

Though we have some broad, consensually validated definitions of words (otherwise verbal communication would be impossible), nevertheless we must be open to the reality that each of us has unique, peculiar meanings and experiences that we bring to words, particularly emotionally charged words like *love*. Hence, the message received will be strongly influenced by those internal references of the receiver.

This would seem to imply that people move from the dynamic experience to the word. In that sense, we project (more than we intend or are aware) our own meanings and associations onto words.

Where the personal experience is somewhat congruent with the consensually validated meaning of the concept, effective communication is likely to occur. That is, the message sent *is* the message received.

Where the personal experience is incongruent with the consensually validated meaning of the concept, communication is likely to be distorted. That is, the message sent is *not* the message received.

Symbols have always been important to the religious community. Most of our traditional symbols are relational in nature. In that sense, they are dynamic, interpersonal and emotionally charged. Because of that, people are even more likely to project onto them their own personal experiences.

Carroll Wise, an early leader in the pastoral care/counseling field, once said: "The only way any formulation of faith can vitally affect personality is for the inner dynamics of personality to become harmonious with the ideas presented."

While some may legitimately contend that the gospel has the power to change those inner dynamics, I do believe that Wise is challenging us to balance our concern about correct theological content by focusing more attention upon the inner dynamics of those to whom we minister. If dynamic learning proceeds from personal experience to the concept and if the major vehicles for such experiences are warm, caring, loving relationships, then the mandate to proclaim the gospel takes on some new and bold dimensions.

Of course, there are dangers to such an emphasis. Attention to the inner dynamics of people can easily lead us to reduce religious faith to one's subjective perceptions. It can lead us to become more interested in people's experience of God than in the nature of God. By oversubjectivizing faith we may wind up supporting a religious faith that is marked by individualism, anti-institutionalism and validated only by the feelings and experiences of that individual at that moment. Such faith can easily lose its authentic, transcendental character, as well as its touch with a historic worshiping community.

In many ways, the chaplain walks between the worlds of theology and psychology, between:

   a faith assumption that claims validity and authenticity for the proclaimed gospel, whether or not it is internally appropriated by the patient; and *a clinical assumption* that asserts that this gospel will have dynamic, functional value for that person only when one's internal realities become consistent with that message.

Or, to put the tension another way, the chaplain knows from clinical experience that there is a vast difference between *being* forgiven and *feeling* forgiven; between *being* loved and *feeling* loved.

To lay hold of both sides of that tension is to allow one's ministry to be informed by both theology and psychology.

Medicine's and Religion's Conflicting Perspectives

While the strong influence of psychology upon ministry has at times fostered tension between the hospital chaplain and the church, conflicting perspectives with regard to suffering have tended to put the chaplain in tension with medicine. Until the era of scientific medicine, suffering was seen essentially as a religious issue. It called upon the sufferer to reflect: "What have I done?" "What does it mean?" "Why did it happen?" "Where is God in it all?" "What must I do?"

The Bible spends much time with the problem of suffering. Though it posits a variety of theories as to the causes of suffering, the Bible's chief value is in helping sufferers to emotionally engage and transcend their suffering.[2]

Jesus' attitude toward suffering was a curious blend of passivity and aggression. On numerous occasions he healed people and no doubt many of his healings were not recorded in the New Testament. But it is apparent that Jesus did not allow his time and energies to be totally consumed with healing diseases, of which there were considerable in his day. Preaching and teaching were fully as important to him.

In fact, nowhere does Jesus suggest that the removal of suffering was his primary mission. Nor does he anywhere hint that the banishment of suffering is anything we could expect as believers. Sin, not suffering was his primary concern. But the healing power was there and on occasion was aggressively employed. His miracles were an active defiance of "enemies": he stilled a storm; he cast out demons; he fed five thousand on morsels; he raised Lazarus from the dead. He fought nature, sickness, hunger, death, head on, and he won.

But that kind of aggressive power was not Jesus' only response to suffering. In his personal suffering he was more passive. He endured it. He submitted, yet transcended it. Through it all, he made abundantly clear that suffering is inevitable. Even more so for his followers.

The early hospices and hospitals — most of which were founded by the newly developed Christian Church — offered more spiritual comfort than they did physical relief. That was the best they could do.

But modern medicine could not write off illness as the working of some obscure, alien force, as an occasion for spiritual reflection. Empirical causes needed to be found. Suffering was an enemy to be conquered, not endured. It had no moral message. It was a vicious power that ravaged and destroyed. Hence, medicine began an aggressive attack upon it. The medical arsenal to do battle grew in numbers and power: potent drugs, antibiotics, surgery, radioactive therapy, chemotherapy, nuclear medicine, electro-convulsive therapy, cardio-pulmonary resuscitation, computerized diagnoses, CAT scans, ultrasound (intraabdominal and intracranial), monitoring, equipment (cardio-monitoring, intraarterial monitoring, pulmonary-venous monitoring). Enemies were uncovered: bacteria, viruses, rickettsia, protozoa, worms.

The aggressiveness paid off. Victories were won, particularly with regard to infectious diseases. True, other allies joined the fight: improved sanitation, purer drinking water, better nutrition, vaccines, higher standards of living, improved housing and working conditions. Little matter which "weapons" did the most. The tide had turned. Smallpox, diphtheria, cholera, tuberculosis, polio, Bright's disease, rheumatic and scarlet fevers and measles were either eliminated or prevented.

One of the unfortunate by-products of the successful war on disease was that it drove a wedge between religion and medicine. There were other losses. There was far more focus on the causes of suffering than upon the sufferer. Human beings were compartmentalized, as were those who treated them. Our views of health and illness became more narrow and physical. Health, in fact, was defined in purely functional terms — as "the absence of illness."

But hospital chaplains were there as the gap between religion and medicine widened. Chaplains willingly joined the fight on disease, though in a lesser rank. But it was hard to fit them in. What could they do to aid the medical enterprise? Encourage people when they got discouraged? Boost their morale? Convince uncooperative patients to cooperate and to accept treatment? The only clear shot the chaplain had was when the patient was dying or dead. Death represented the failure of medicine. It was a battle lost. But by and large the chaplain's role was an accommodating one. What else could a chaplain do in a setting which defined sickness in strictly physical terms?

It was impossible to quantify the chaplain's contribution. What difference did it really make in the functional recovery of a patient to know that one's sins were forgiven, that the forces of evil are submissive to God's ultimate will, that the sting of death has been removed in the resurrection of Jesus Christ?

This was the chaplain's dilemma in the thirties, forties and early fifties: seeking acceptance in the clinical world but not really finding a relevant role that was respected in and by that world.

As we reached the sixties and seventies some changes began to occur that impacted both chaplaincy and medicine. After those early medical victories, new illnesses replaced the old, many of them harder to pin down and destroy: heart attacks, hypertension, depression, addictions, accidents, emotional and physical violence. These new illnesses seemed more related to phenomena such as stress, pressure, life-style, relationships. Now the battleground was not so clear-cut, the enemy not so neatly defined, the medical arsenal not nearly so potent.

Though the new battle brought frustrations and fewer victories than before, it caused the medical world to rethink its concepts of health and illness. Medical professionals and hospitals began to think more wholistically. At Lutheran General Hospital, this rethinking produced a definition of human ecology: "The understanding and care of human beings as whole persons in light of their relationships to God, to themselves, their families and society in which they live." This broad view saw illness as a complex interaction between the biological-psychological-social-mental-spiritual forces within persons, as well as the interplay of heredity, environment, decisions, life-styles, diet, exercise, values, faith meanings and commitments.

In many ways these new developments were not really new. Indeed, the Latin word *casus* (from which comes English, "case") meant "a fall out of harmony." Illness has always been a disharmony on many fronts. To explore and to treat those various dimensions of disharmony within each person and family is the recaptured task of today's hospital. It is a rediscovery task that needs to be seriously engaged if we are to be as effective in this "second war" as we were in the first.

Just as illness is multidimensional, so — we are increasingly coming to see — are the resources for health. There are physical, social, emotional, intellectual, spiritual capacities and strengths within people, which need to be mobilized and channeled. There are family systems and social units that are sources of healing. In addition, patients are now being seen as active participants in their own health, as we continue to discover the vital links between habits, life-styles, beliefs, values and health.

The approaches to health care are broadening. There has also come an increased recognition of the need for interdisciplinary understanding and interaction. As illness is now seen in more complex terms, so has followed the recognition that no one profession or method or service can independently or exclusively meet all the forces of illness. Hospitals today seek to foster a milieu in which many professions have the opportunity to employ their own unique skills, perspectives, and goals in the care of people, but where each discipline is also charged with responsibility to assess critically its contribution to optimal patient care. In many sectors pastoral care has won a place of relevance and respect in and by the clinical world.

But there are still tensions. Perhaps at no point is the chaplain's role seen as more divergent from medicine than in this very area of disease and treatment. Put succinctly: *the chaplain's role is not to explain, cure, or eliminate disease.*

The chaplain seeks only to engage the sufferer. In so doing, the chaplain harbors no illusions about the banishment of suffering. Indeed, from the Babylonian captivity to the crucifixion, to the Domitian persecutions, to the bubonic plague, to Auschwitz and Hiroshima, on and on it goes. Suffering has not lessened. It has only taken different forms.

The chaplain's theological perspective breeds cynicism about any medical efforts to banish suffering. Indeed, the chaplain has a prophetic word of caution to the medical community, namely, *that we not give suffering more than its due.*[3] That caution would seek to remind that community that suffering is not infinite. Like us, like death, like angels and principalities, it is a creature. Like all creatures, it is subservient to the Creator. The chaplain knows that suffering does end — by healing or by death. That prophetic word does not deny suffering its reality, but it refuses to concede its ultimacy. The chaplain's is a prophetic word that grants to suffering power and devastation, but not the last word in life and history. God is the last word. And that word is the chaplain's word to the medical community.

Eugene Peterson puts it well: "The task of pastoral care is to join the sufferer, to enter the pain, to engage the absurdity, to descend into hell . . . not to minimize or to mitigate the suffering," but to help the sufferer to put the suffering in perspective.[4]

Such a role certainly is at variance with the role and mission of the medical enterprise. A touch of irony is in that pastoral role, for the chaplain represents the God who could banish human suffering in the blink of an eye. Yet, all the chaplain can do, as God's emissary, is to bring a companionship to the sufferer.

Yet it is a special companionship, to a specific sufferer, at a specific moment in history. God's deliverance is always concrete and specific: the Exodus from Egypt, the theophany at Sinai, the conquest of Canaan, the enthronement on Zion, the birth at Bethlehem, the crucifixion at Calvary, the empty tomb — the chaplain at the bedside. That's how concrete and specific God's engagement is with suffering people.

However, the chaplain's prophetic word to the medical establishment is not a cry for masochism, not a plea that humanity acquiesce to the devastations of suffering. Suffering is an enemy, rarely a friend. We chaplains join the relentless crusade to limit its power. But that can never be the chaplain's primary mission, that is, if the chaplain remains faithful to the source of ministry. For deep down the chaplain knows that suffering will prevail and that it can be redemptive, for "suffering produces endurance, and endurance produces character, and character produces hope and hope does not disappoint us" (Rom 5:3-4).

Conclusion

The chaplain walks between two powerful, influential worlds: religion and medicine. The chaplain identifies with both worlds; yet does not feel entirely at home in either. Chaplains are an enigma to both worlds: medicine does not consider them "medical enough" and questions their relevance; the church often does not consider them "pastoral enough" and questions their identity. But the fact is that despite the tensions and enigmas, the hospital chaplain is very much committed to both worlds and is a vital link between them.

It is more than coincidental that as hospital chaplaincy has grown in numbers and influence in the sixties, seventies, and early eighties that religion and medicine now find themselves in more serious engagement than at any time in the twentieth century.

Though it might seem contradictory, the hospital chaplain is also a reminder that the worlds of religion and medicine are and must remain distinct. For while those two worlds need engagement with, they also need separation from, one another if both are to preserve their distinct and vital missions. So, it can be expected and hoped that the hospital chaplain will always walk in two worlds.

NOTES

1. Thomas Droegge, *Faith Passages and Patterns* (Philadelphia: Fortress Press, 1983), pp. 12-13.

2. Daniel J. Simundson, *Faith Under Fire: Biblical Interpretations of Suffering* (Minneapolis: Augsburg Publishing House, 1980), p. 144.

3. Eugene Peterson, *Five Smooth Stones for Pastoral Work* (Atlanta: John Knox Press, 1980), p. 101.

4. Ibid., p. 110.

3

Change in Perceived Need, Value and Role of Hospital Chaplains

RAYMOND G. CAREY

The previous chapter outlined the philosophical, theological, and practical issues that touch the chaplain's efforts to work between the worlds of religion and medicine in the common goal of bringing "wholeness" to patients.

But what has been the nature and extent of success of these efforts? How has the medical staff perceived the chaplain? As help or interference? Do nurses see chaplains as enhancing efforts to create a healing environment on a hospital unit? What do patients want and actually receive from a hospital chaplain? Are chaplains agreed on their role priorities?

In 1971 (when the field of evaluation research was just beginning in the wake of the Government Accounting Office's effort to see how Medicare and Medicaid money was being spent, and before the Evaluation Research Society was formed), Lutheran General Hospital commissioned a study to try to answer these questions. The results of this study were published in a report entitled "Hospital Chaplains: Who Needs Them?" (Carey, 1974). Some key findings were:

> The availability of chaplains was highly valued by patients and received an even stronger endorsement from physicians and nurses.
>
> Age and religious preference of patients were important variables in the assessing value patients placed on chaplaincy.
>
> The policy of assigning chaplains to care for all patients on a unit regardless of religious preference was supported.
>
> The value that chaplains placed on various aspects of their ministry differed substantially from the value system of patients, indicating that role communication needed to be improved.

In the decade that followed, the report assumed added significance when third-party payers and Medicare representatives challenged the hospital's use of money from room charges to underwrite the services of a very large Division of Pastoral Care. (This report was successfully used in the response to those efforts to challenge reimbursement.)

The decision to repeat the evaluation of the chaplaincy services in 1981 was prompted by both internal and external reasons. Internally, the Division of Pastoral Care wanted to learn whether there had been any changes in the attitudes and values of patients and hospital staff toward pastoral care during the intervening decade. In addition, new factors were present: resident physicians were now a part of the health care delivery team; women were a sizable minority of the pastoral care staff; and pastoral care was giving new emphasis to certain roles (e.g., as ethical resources, a prophetic role toward the hospital administration, solidifying its relationship to community clergy). Externally, the Division of Pastoral Care anticipated that increasing pressure would be put upon chief executive officers to cut budgets wherever possible, especially for nonrevenue-producing services. Such pressure could result in efforts to reduce pastoral care staff or services unless solid and up-to-date data were available to demonstrate the value of chaplains to patients and hospital staff. (In December 1982 the hospital faced a challenge of a portion of its Clinical Pastoral Education program by the Health Care Financial Administration. The hospital's appeal was upheld by the H.C.F.A. board.)

The specific objectives of the 1981 study were to answer the following questions:

> What is the overall value of chaplains to patients, physicians, and nurses?

> What specific services do patients, physicians, and nurses value most?

> How does the role definition of chaplains differ from the expectations of patients, physicians and nurses?

> What major roles of the chaplains can be identified?

> To what extent have role expectations and role values changed over the decade?

The same basic design with some modifications was used in the 1981 study as was used in 1971. The questionnaire listed 19 items that might be considered aspects of chaplain ministry (table 3 below). Respondents were asked about *role expectation* (i.e., whether or not they felt each item was a part of the work of a chaplain) and *role value* (i.e., the extent to which it was important to them as a patient, physician, nurse to have a chaplain provide the help or service described). This distinction was made because it was suspected that most repondents would feel that saying good things about chaplains was expected of them. Providing the role expectation rating allowed respondents to say that they expected chaplains to fill a role (the socially desirable response), but the role value rating allowed them to report that fulfilling that role may not be of great personal value to the respondent. This technique worked effectively in both the 1971 and 1981 surveys.

One hundred and twenty patients were sampled from 12 units. To qualify as a respondent, a patient had to have been in the hospital for at least 24 hours. In addition, the head nurse of each unit had to give assurance that the patients were able to be interviewed without the risk of causing them discomfort or distress.

Six nurses were sampled from the same 12 units, although the head nurses were always included in the sample (total = 72).

Fifty physicians were sampled from the Divisions of Internal Medicine, Family Practice, Surgery.

All permanent staff chaplains, one-year Clinical Pastoral Education residents, and C.P.E. quarter students were included in the chaplain group.

In summary, the same four respondent groups were surveyed as in 1971; namely, patients, physicians, nurses, and chaplains. The description of these four groups is presented in tables 1 and 2 below. The response rate ranged from 90% for patients to 100% for chaplains.

The profiles of the four groups were substantially the same as in 1971. However, there were some differences:

> *Patients.* In 1981 there were 42% of patients in the sample over 60 years of age, as compared to 20% in 1971. This is representative of the overall patient population and reflects the demographic change in the community. From the standpoint of religious affiliation, the 1981 patient sample included a small percentage (5%) of patients who professed Eastern religions and a smaller percentage of Lutheran patients. Only 34% of the patients in the 1981 sample reported monthly church attendance. Data on church attendance was not available for the 1971 study.

Chaplains. All staff chaplains and student chaplains were again invited to participate in the study. In 1981, 11 (28%) of the respondents were women, as compared to one woman in 1971. The number of staff chaplains increased from 10 to 26 during the decade.

Nurses. The profile of nurses was much the same as in 1981: 62% were under 30 years of age; 35% were Catholic and 36% were Protestant. However, in 1981, 10% claimed to have no religious preference and 8% belonged to Eastern religions, as compared to only 1% with no religious preference and no affliliates of Eastern religions in 1971.

Physicians. The main difference in the 1981 sample of physicians was the inclusion of 8 (17%) residents in the sample. The average age of the sample was slightly older in 1981. With respect to religious preference, 26% of the total were Protestant, 36% Catholic, and 34% Jewish.

1981 Survey Results

The results of the survey are examined in five main areas.

Perceived Need

To get a feeling of the overall value of chaplain availability the patients and staff were asked two similar questions: "What is the importance of having a chaplain of the SAME faith (denomination) available to the patients at all times?" and "What is the importance of having a chaplain of SOME faith available at all times?"

The responses were very similar to those in 1971. First, only about a third of each group felt it was of great importance to have a chaplain of the SAME faith (denomination) as the patient available at all times. Second, a higher percentage of nurses and physicians than patients endorsed the importance of having a chaplain of SOME faith available. However, while the percentage of patients responding "of great importance" to the second question increased from 40% in 1971 to 56% in 1981, the percentage of physicians so responding decreased from 76% to 62% and that of nurses from 87% to 83%.

Role Expectations

As was previously stated, the main reason for distinguishing between role expectations and role value was to address the tendency for respondents to give socially desirable answers. The technique was successful insofar as all respondent groups gave every item higher role expectation scores than role value scores. To check on the care with which respondents answered on each role item, two items (12 and 13) were retained from 1971 that were expected to receive very little support as a chaplain responsibility. The results were as expected (see table 3 below).

Results show that patients do not view the role of the chaplain to be as extensive as do the hospital staff and the chaplains themselves. For example, a majority of patients do not believe it is the chaplain's job to be "a resource to physicians and nurses on ethics issues" (item 6), to conduct classes for "medical or nursing students on subjects of pastoral concern" (item 7), "to help hospital employees with their personal or work problems" (item 12), or "to confront hospital administration for departing from hospital philosophy" (item 18), while the majority of hospital staff and chaplain respondents see these activities as part of the chaplain's responsibility.

Role Values

Of the 19 role items presented in the questionnaire, a majority of patients placed "high" value on 4 items, a majority of physicians placed "high" value on 9 items, a majority of nurses placed a "high" value on 10 items, and a majority of chaplains placed "high" value on 11 items (table 3 below).

With respect to the hierarchy of values, the value systems of patients, nurses, and physicians were very similar, while the value system of chaplains differed from the other groups on some items. As in 1971 the patients, nurses, and physicians placed highest value on helping the patients face death (item 9), comforting patients' relatives (item 10), and administering the sacraments (item 8).

However, the chaplains rated the witness role (item 1) and helping patients cope with fear (item 4) as the roles valued most highly, while these roles were ranked fourth to sixth by the other groups. Chaplains ranked administering the sacraments and conducting worship services considerably lower than the other groups. With respect to the "team role," 73% of nurses and 95% of chaplains placed high value on having chaplains work with nurses and physicians as part of a team, while only 47% of physicians and 30% of patients ranked this item as having high value. Finally, a majority of physicians placed high value on having chaplains confront administration when policies or practices seemed inconsistent with the hospital's philosophy of human ecology (item 18), while only a minority of other respondents did so.

Attending physicians see more value in chaplains than do resident physicians. The median percentage of "high" ratings given by attending physicians to the 19 items was 56% compared to a median percentage of 25% given by residents. However, the residents strongly endorsed four chaplain activities: helping patients cope with fears and anxieties, administering the sacraments, helping patients face death, and comforting patients' relatives at the time of serious illness. Residents were clearly not supportive of having chaplains consult with doctors and nurses as part of a team working for total patient care.

Patients were divided according to religious affiliation, age, and gender, but few differences of notable importance appeared.

Nurses were divided according to religious affiliation, age, and tenure, but no notable differences appeared.

Chaplains were divided according to religious affiliation, staff versus students, age, and gender. Staff chaplains put greater emphasis on counseling patients on ethical issues (item 5) and on being a resource for physicians and nurses (item 6) than did student chaplains. Older chaplains put more emphasis on visiting patients the night before an operation (item 3) than did younger chaplains. Chaplains in the 30 to 39 year-old age group put much less emphasis on praying with patients (item 16), confronting hospital administration (item 18), and working with the community clergy (item 19) than did the other three age groups. Women chaplains put more emphasis on praying privately for individual patients (item 15) than did male patients. There were few other differences of note.

Five Major Roles

When the 19 items listed as possible chaplain activities were factor analyzed, they were reduced to five major roles: comforter, liturgist, witness, resource person, and counselor (table 4 below). The item ratings of all respondents were recalculated to provide ratings for these 5 major roles (table 5 below). As can readily be seen in table 5, the comforter role was the most highly valued by all 4 respondent groups and the counselor role was least valued. The group mean (averages) for all groups were almost identical for nurses, physicians, and chaplains, while the patient mean (average) score was considerably lower. This latter finding supports the results reported earlier.

Selected Issues of Interest

More than two-thirds of the patients said they would appreciate a visit by a chaplain, their own local clergy, or both. However, only 28% said it was of great importance to have the hospital notify their parish of their hospitalization.

Two thirds of the physicians preferred chaplains who were clergy or religious, while a slight majority of the other groups had no preference for lay or religious chaplains as long as they were qualified.

Although patients were selected only if they had been hospitalized for at least 24 hours, 37% said they had not been visited as yet. However, of those who had been visited, 81% were pleased with the chaplain's ministry. Ninety percent of nurses and 78% of physicians also said they were pleased with the ministry of the chaplains.

Implications of the Findings

The 1981 survey results have implications in three main areas.

Chaplain Service

Are chaplains providing a valuable service to the hosptial? Yes, emphatically. A solid majority of patients and an overwhelming majority of nurses and physicians report that it is of great importance to have a chaplain of some faith (denomination) available to the patient at all times. The overwhelming majority of respondents also say they were pleased with the ministry of the chaplains. The chaplain's role as a comforter (table 3 below, items 4, 9, 10) was the most important to all respondent groups.

Value System

In what way is the value system of chaplains different from patients, nurses, and physicians? Chaplains view their witness role (table 3 below, items 1, 15, 16, 17) as more important than their liturgist role (table 3, items 9 and 11), while these priorities are reversed for patients, nurses, and physicians.

The majority of chaplains put high value on being a resource to nurses and physicians on ethical issues, while only a minority of nurses and physicians do so (table 3, item 6).

The majority of physicians would like to see chaplains confront administration when policies or practices seem inconsistent with hospital philosophy, while the majority of chaplains do not see this as a high value.

Further Issues

Issues to be addressed as a result of the study include the following:

Medical-ethical. Since medical-ethical issues have become so prominent in our society today, how can a chaplain's role in such issues become more visible? Clearly, chaplains feel the need for addressing these issues intensely and, in general, are better equipped by education and training to address them than many other professionals.

The Division of Pastoral Care at Lutheran General has taken two meaningful steps toward involving the chaplain in ethical issues since this study was published: first, it has retained a consulting ethicist to help define and articulate a role; and, second, a Human Values Forum, chaired by the Division of Pastoral Care, has been developed to study moral-ethical issues that confront the hospital and to conduct seminars and symposia.

Prophetic Role. Should the Division of Pastoral Care assume the responsibility of what might be called a prophetic role in monitoring apparent violations of hospital philosophy or policy by hospital staff or administration? If so, what organizational avenue should be developed to facilitate a meaningful contribution from the Division of Pastoral Care?

Why is it chaplains value an ethical role with physicians and nurses (51%), but less so with patients (36%) and less than a confrontational role with administration (43%)? Clearly, the latter puts the chaplain in a more controversial, prophetic role and could possibly pit the chaplain against those toward whom he or she is accountable, namely, administration. The Human Values Forum is now establishing ethical criteria by which to evaluate consistency of hospital policy with those principles. But that is evaluating policy, not administrative action.

Need for Initiating Patient Contact. Chaplains must deal with the reality of low expectations and high satisfaction. That is, about one-third of patient respondents placed value on a chaplain's visit during their hospitalization, yet 81% expressed satisfaction with ministry when the chaplain did visit. This suggests that chaplains must take the initiative since patients are not likely to request visits. Most chaplains would agree that taking initiative is very difficult. Chaplains prefer responding to patient or staff initiative (see chap. 6 below).

It would appear that the parish pastor faces the same task of taking initiative with hospitalized parishioners. While it was not a major focus of the 1981 study, only 28% of patients placed high value on having their parish pastors/priests notified of their hospitalization. Chaplains and local clergy might profit by addressing this problem together.

Team Role. The chaplain obviously values inclusion on the team more than the other respondents do. Why? Is that the chaplain's insecurity? Do others prize the confidential/confessional role and not want that compromised? Or is it simply that others fail to see the relationship of faith/values to their medical care? Is this issue important to the chaplain because of a fear that religion (and the chaplain) not be compartmentalized?

Visibility. How can the demonstrated value of pastoral care be given better visibility both within the hospital and to outside bodies, such as, government agencies and third-party payers? As a first step, evaluation research needs to be continually updated as roles and conditions change. Research also needs to be replicated in different settings to demonstrate the commonality of the findings.

Table 1. Description of Respondents: Patients and Chaplains

Descriptor	*Patients*		*Chaplains*	
Sample Size	*Number*	*%*	*Number*	*%*
Number of surveys distributed	120	—	39	—
Completed surveys	109	90%	39	100%
Gender				
Male	39	36%	27	69%
Female	63	58	11	28
No answer	7	6	1	3
Age				
Under 20	0	0%	0	0%
20 to 29	16	15	5	13
30 to 39	18	17	9	23
40 to 49	10	9	16	41
50 to 59	14	13	8	21
60 or over	46	42	0	0
No answer	5	5	1	3
Religious preference				
Lutheran	17	16%	11	28%
Other Protestant	26	24	18	46
Catholic	37	34	8	21
Jewish	9	8	2	5
Other	5	5	0	0
None	11	10	0	0
No answer	4	4	0	0

Descriptor	Patients		Chaplains	
Frequency of worship	Number	%	Number	%
Weekly	22	20%	—	—
1–3 times per month	15	14	—	—
A few times a year	32	29	—	—
Rarely or never	30	28	—	—
No answer	10	9	—	—
Marital Status				
Single	6	6%	—	—
Married	75	69	—	—
Widow/er	16	16	—	—
Divorced or separated	7	6	—	—
No answer	4	4	—	—
Length of stay				
Under 8 days	61	56%	—	—
8 to 14 days	25	23	—	—
Over 14 days	18	17	—	—
No answer	5	5	—	—
Chaplain appointment				
Staff	—	—	26	67%
Resident	—	—	6	15
Quarter student	—	—	7	18

Table 2. Description of Respondents: Nurses and Physicians

Descriptor	Nurses		Physicians	
Sample Size	Number	%	Number	%
Number of surveys distributed	72	—	50	—
Completed surveys	71	99%	47	94%
Gender				
Male	0	0%	42	89%
Female	69	97	2	4
No answer	2	3	3	6
Age				
Under 20	0	0%	0	0%
20 to 29	45	63	4	8
30 to 39	13	18	14	30
40 to 49	7	10	13	28
50 to 59	4	6	16	34
60 or over	0	0	0	0
No answer	2	3	0	0

Descriptor	Nurses		Physicians	
Religious Preference	*Number*	%	*Number*	%
Lutheran	13	18%	5	11%
Other Protestant	13	18	7	15
Catholic	25	35	15	32
Jewish	2	3	16	34
Other	6	8	2	4
None	7	10	2	4
No answer	5	7	0	0
Years at LGH				
Under 1	19	27%	—	—
1 to 2	12	17	—	—
2 or more	34	48	—	—
No answer	6	8	—	—
Nurse degree				
R.N.	56	79%	—	—
L.P.N.	8	11	—	—
No answer	7	10	—	—
Physician specialty				
Medicine	—	—	14	30%
Family practice	—	—	10	21
Obstetrics and Gynecology	—	—	7	15
Surgery	—	—	9	19
Psychiatry	—	—	7	15
Physician appointment				
Attending staff	—	—	39	83%
Resident	—	—	8	17

Table 3. ROLE VALUE: Percentage of Each Respondent Group Placing High Personal Value on Possible Chaplain Activities

Chaplain Activity	Patients (n = 109) %H (R)*	Nurses (n = 71) %H (R)*	Physicians (n = 47) %H (R)*	Chaplains (n = 39) %H (R)*
1. To be present with patients and/or family in time of crisis as a *witness* of God's love and concern.	50 (4)	84 (4)	62 (6)	97 (1)
2. To visit each patient *at least once* while hospitalized.	36 (10)	38 (13)	45 (11)	24 (18)

Chaplain Activity	Patients (n = 109) %H (R)*	Nurses (n = 71) %H (R)*	Physicians (n = 47) %H (R)*	Chaplains (n = 39) %H (R)*
3. To visit patients the night before an *operation*.	42 (7)	58 (9)	30 (15)	54 (9)
4. To help patients cope with *fears* and *anxieties* resulting from illness.	46 (5)	65 (6)	62 (6)	97 (1)
5. To counsel *patients on ethical issues* (rightness or wrongness of actions).	15 (16)	16 (18)	30 (15)	36 (16)
6. To be a resource for *physicians* and *nurses* on ethical issues.	15 (16)	32 (15)	40 (13)	51 (10)
7. To conduct *lectures* or *classes* for medical or nursing *students* on subjects of pastoral concern.	13 (18)	28 (16)	34 (17)	31 (17)
8. To administer the *Sacraments* to patients upon request.	67 (1)	86 (3)	94 (1)	69 (8)
9. To help the patient face *death*.	66 (3)	87 (2)	85 (2)	92 (4)
10. To comfort the patient's relatives at the time of serious illness or death.	67 (1)	97 (1)	85 (2)	87 (6)
11. To provide *worship* services in the hospital.	42 (7)	62 (7)	66 (5)	50 (12)
12. To help hospital employees with their personal and work problems.	16 (15)	24 (17)	21 (18)	47 (13)
13. To handle patient's *questions* and complaints about the hospital administration, physicians or nurses.	15 (16)	14 (19)	6 (19)	8 (19)
14. To consult with doctors and nurses as part of a *team* working for total patient care.	30 (13)	73 (5)	47 (10)	95 (3)

Chaplain Activity	Patients (n = 109) %H (R)*	Nurses (n = 71) %H (R)*	Physicians (n = 47) %H (R)*	Chaplains (n = 39) %H (R)*
15. To pray *privately* for individual patients.	43 (6)	35 (14)	36 (14)	46 (14)
16. To pray *with* individual patients.	41 (9)	61 (8)	45 (11)	78 (7)
17. To help patients with their *own* efforts to pray.	35 (12)	52 (10)	55 (9)	89 (5)
18. To confront *hospital administration* when policies or practice seem inconsistent with the philosophy of Human Ecology.	18 (14)	44 (12)	57 (8)	43 (15)
19. To work with *community clergy* in their ministry to hospitalized parishioners.	36 (10)	46 (11)	70 (4)	51 (10)
Median Percentage	41	58	55	54
Most important items and percentage selecting them (%): First	# 9 (11%)	# 1 (25%)	# 4 (21%)	# 1 (69%)
Second	#10 (10%)	# 4 (16%) #10 (16%)	# 1 (13%) # 9 (13%)	# 4 (15%)

*Percentage "High" answers.
(R) = rank order

Table 4. Items Making Up Five Major Chaplain Roles

Chaplain Role	Item Number and Role Statement
Comforter	4. To help patients cope with *fears* and *anxieties* resulting from illness. 9. To help the patient face *death*. 10. To comfort the patient's *relatives* at the time of serious illness or death.
Liturgist	8. To administer the *Sacraments* to patients upon request. 11. To provide worship *services* in the hospital.

Chaplain Role	Item Number and Role Statement
Witness	1. To be present with patients and/or families in time of crisis as a *witness* of God's love and concern. 15. To pray *privately* for individual patients. 16. To pray *with* individual patients. 17. To help patients with their *own* efforts to pray.
Resource Person	6. To be a resource for *physicians* and *nurses* on *ethical issues*. 7. To conduct *lectures* or *classes* for medical or nursing *students* on subjects of pastoral concern. 14. To consult with doctors and nurses as part of a *team* working for total patient care. 18. To confront *hospital administration* when policies or practice seem inconsistent with the philosophy of Human Ecology. 19. To work with *community clergy* in their ministry to hospitalized parishioners.
Counselor	2. To *visit* each patient *at least once* while hospitalized. 3. To visit patients the night before an *operation*. 5. To counsel *patients* on *ethical* issues (rightness or wrongness of actions). 12. To help *hospital employees* with their personal and work problems. 13. To handle patient's *questions* and *complaints* about the hospital administration, physicians or nurses.

Table 5. Mean Value Assigned by Each Respondent Group to Five Major Roles of Chaplain

Chaplain Role	Patients	Nurses	Physicians	Chaplain	Overall Role Mean
Comforter	2.60 (1)	2.80 (1)	2.80 (1)	2.90 (1)	2.78
Liturgist	2.42 (2)	2.70 (2)	2.78 (2)	2.47 (3)	2.59
Witness	2.29 (3)	2.60 (3)	2.42 (4)	2.70 (2)	2.50
Resource Person	1.83 (4)	2.36 (4)	2.45 (3)	2.47 (3)	2.28
Counselor	1.80 (5)	2.00 (5)	1.90 (5)	2.14 (5)	1.96
Overall Group Mean	2.19	2.49	2.47	2.50	

Note: These means have been standardized to achieve equivalent ranges for all ratings. Lowest value possible equals 1.00, highest possible, 3.00. Rank order in parentheses.

4

The Hospital Chaplain: One Role, Many Functions

LAWRENCE E. HOLST

"It's no big emergency," the nurse intoned, "but we could sure use you."
The plea came from a surgical nurse to a duty chaplain. The reason for
the call was a highly agitated female patient who was scheduled for a
potentially serious surgical procedure the following day.

A quick glance at the patient's chart revealed that Mrs. Iverson was
sixty-four years old, a widow, a Lutheran with no specific congregation
identified and with a diagnosis of suspected cancer of the colon. Moments later the chaplain found himself at the patient's bedside.

CHAPLAIN. Mrs. Iverson, I'm Chaplain Holman, a chaplain at the hospital. I know that you are going to surgery tomorrow and your nurse
suggested that I stop by.

PATIENT. Oh, thank you, chaplain. I guess I haven't made it very easy
for the nurses. I'm a bit upset. I've never been to surgery, have you?

CHAPLAIN. Yes, some years ago. It's understandable that you'd be
upset.

PATIENT. But I shouldn't be. I know I'm in good hands. I have faith in
my doctors and I have faith in God. But this whole thing has gone on
so long. I hope I haven't waited too long.

CHAPLAIN. You mean waited too long to come into the hospital?

PATIENT. Yes. I had this bleeding and I didn't say anything. I'm alone,
you know. I didn't want to bother Dorothy with this. She's my daughter. She's got her hands full with her five children. I already feel that
I've been a nuisance to them.

CHAPLAIN. So, your fear is that you delayed going to the doctor, and you
feel you've overburdened your daughter.

PATIENT. [on the verge of tears]. I have to depend on my daughter to take
me everywhere. I don't drive. Everything is happening so fast. I was

never sick when I was younger and had a husband. That's when I should have gotten sick. When I had someone to take care of me. Instead, I took care of my husband.

CHAPLAIN. It doesn't seem fair, does it?

PATIENT. Well, do you think it is fair? Tomorrow they're going to cut me open and then they'll have to find a place for me. I'd be better off if I just died. Then everyone could just go on with their lives.

CHAPLAIN. [just nodded, but remained silent].

PATIENT. Oh, I'll be all right. I just have to grow up and have more faith, that's all. I'll bet you've seen a lot of sick people tonight.

CHAPLAIN. [again, just nodded].

PATIENT. You'd think at my age I wouldn't be such a coward, but I don't know what I'm going to do. I can't seem to care for myself anymore, and it all falls on Dorothy.

CHAPLAIN. You feel very much alone, don't you, Mrs. Iverson?

PATIENT. [just stared out the window]. I must sound awful to you, chaplain. I'm sure you've got lots of other patients to see. I'm taking up too much of your time.

CHAPLAIN. You feel you're imposing on me too, Mrs. Iverson, but you're not.

PATIENT. [no response, just looked away].

CHAPLAIN. Would you like to talk more about this?

PATIENT. [abruptly and coldly]. About what?

CHAPLAIN. About your fears of surgery, about your concerns of being so dependent upon others.

PATIENT. [brief pause]. What's the use of talking about it? It doesn't help. Aren't you a chaplain? Don't you have any encouragement for people like me? I don't understand all your questions. I feel worse than when you came in.

CHAPLAIN. [somewhat anxiously]. It does seem as though you've been more frustrated than helped by my visit.

PATIENT. [now very agitated]. You're right. I'm telling you I'm old and old people are in the way. We should move over and let the young people go on through. God should just take me. What else is there to say?

CHAPLAIN. Mrs. Iverson, I hear your words and I think I catch many of your feelings. It's OK to feel as you do, it's understandable. I'm sure God understands and accepts your feelings.

PATIENT. No, it isn't OK. I'm not doing myself or anyone any good. I shouldn't feel this way. I know it and God knows it.

CHAPLAIN. That must make you feel even more lonely.

PATIENT. Chaplain, I'm fine. I'll get through this. I don't feel that you're helping me. It's not what I need right now.

The visit ended a few awkward moments later, on a frustrating note for both the patient and the chaplain.

Regardless of how one would evaluate the interviewing skills of the chaplain, this brief preoperative visit reveals a disparity in the expectations of the patient and the chaplain, and even the nurse. The patient wanted assurances that her troublesome feelings were under control; the nurse sought composure for an agitated preoperative patient; the chaplain wanted the patient to face and accept the turbulent feelings that were gnawing at her. All were legitimate expectations.

In fact, all three of them had a common goal: to help Mrs. Iverson better prepare herself for the very demanding surgical experience that awaited her. It was at the level of *means* that the disparate expectations surfaced. The means employed by the chaplain were confusing to the patient.

Chaplain Holman's knowledge of psychodynamics supplied him with skills that prompted him to behave in ways that were confusing to the patient. He wanted to help Mrs. Iverson face and accept her strong feelings about aging, dependency, abandonment, and delaying medical care. She wanted help in suppressing, not provoking, such feelings. As a result, an impasse resulted where the patient felt deprived and the chaplain felt thwarted.

It appears that the patient was also disillusioned by the chaplain's failure to offer encouragement and to employ familiar, religious language and rituals. She had a religious identity and made frequent references to God and faith. The perceived underutilization of traditional religious resources is a sore point for hospital chaplains. Sometimes this underutilization is due to a chaplain's negligence and inability. Sometimes it is due to an unfamiliarity with the patient and to an honest conflict in role models.

Patients who come out of a parish involvement bring with them "a parish pastor role model." This is understandable since that has been their primary exposure to pastors. That role model tends to see the pastor in an active, dispensing mode. Parishioners have seen their pastor / priest / rabbi administrate the congregation, lead worship, preach and teach God's word, recruit, mobilize, direct. They have seen their clergy initiate, take charge. They have found themselves in a responsive receiving mode. There is, then, the understandable tendency to project that familiar role model onto the hospital chaplain (see chap. 3 above).

However, because of the context, the unfamiliarity with the patient, the clinical training and skills of the chaplain, the hospital chaplain's role model tends to be that of a facilitator, rather than a dispenser. It is a more passive role model. This difference is often confusing to patients and may fail to meet their needs and expectations. When this occurs, the patient (as with Mrs. Iverson) feels underserved; the chaplain (as with Chaplain Holman) feels underutilized.

In our presurgical scenario, Chaplain Holman was convinced that Mrs. Iverson could be better prepared, emotionally and spiritually, by honestly facing her anger, fears, and guilt. To put a cap on these feelings, to cover that dark, shadowy side, might provide momentary relief but possibly at the risk of later psychic pain. For, as Chaplain Holman's clinical understandings informed him, feelings that are denied are not thereby destroyed.

It appeared to the chaplain that the patient was struggling with two self-images: her "real self," which included raw, primitive, intense emotions that were frightening and painful; and her "ideal self" which could not admit to such feelings. Without realizing it, Mrs. Iverson was appealing to Chaplain Holman to support her ideal self, one she considered more acceptable to God whose judgment she now feared and whose protection she now coveted. The chaplain's goal was to help the patient get more in touch with her real self and to help her trust God's acceptance of that "shadowy side."

One could argue that the chaplain was correct in his analysis but wrong in his timing. In view of the pending surgical trauma, support and suppression might have been preferred short-term strategies. However, the use of this preoperative conversation between chaplain and patient is not to evaluate the clinical skills and judgment of the chaplain, but rather to see through it the divergent expectations of both the patient and the chaplain—expectations that are not uncommon.

Pastoral Care: What Is It?

What is it that Chaplain Holman was seeking to provide Patient Iverson? The answer, of course, is pastoral care. To understand what pastoral care is, look at the two words themselves.

Care is something that is universally human. It is going on in every moment of human existence. No one takes care of oneself in every respect.

Care is mutual—one who gives it also receives it. Everyone is at some point in time both a giver and receiver of care.

Care is both attitude and action. It is being positively disposed toward another. Care is seeking the best interest of another. But it is also allowing that disposition, or attitude, to issue in concrete acts. Certainly, chaplains do not have a monopoly on care in a hospital. Care is expected of all people who work there.

Care is *pastoral* when its power and focus are seen to be beyond self, beyond human. Paul Tillich expressed its uniqueness as "a helping encounter in the dimension of ultimate concern." He says that "its function is to communicate the power of the Divine which is eternal and which conquers all forces of non-being." "It is the power," Tillich concludes, "which mediates the courage to accept finitude and the anxiety of creatureliness."[1]

Hence, care that is universal becomes uniquely pastoral when it helps to direct others to the source of life and power, to that which alone is infinite and eternal.

Pastoral Care: One Role

It is my contention that *all pastoral care has a basic, primary, definable, fundamental role.* By role is meant a basic task or purpose as determined by one's office, profession, or position. Role is a combination of external (imposed) and internal (self) expectations. In the case of a hospital chaplain, that role is determined by one's religious tradition, by one's context, by one's skills, and by the needs of those who receive that ministry.

I would define that basic, fundamental role of pastoral care as *the attempt to help others, through words, acts, and relationships, to experience as fully as possible the reality of God's presence and love in their lives.*

Pastoral Care: Many Functions

That defined pastoral role is carried out by the hospital chaplain through a variety of functions. By function is meant the ways and means whereby role is implemented.

This leads me to a second contention that *the major controversies about hospital chaplaincy have more to do with functions than they have to do with role.*

To elaborate on this thesis, it is helpful to draw upon two terms employed by Thomas Oden, "implicit" and "explicit."[2] These were used by him to describe God's self-disclosure in the context of a psychotherapeutic relationship. For my purposes here I have substituted the terms "overt" and "covert" to describe two general types of pastoral functions within the context of hospital chaplaincy.

Some pastoral functions are "overtly pastoral" in that they are performed specifically, distinctly and, in many cases, exclusively by an ordained pastor. Such functions include worship leadership, preaching, administration of the sacraments, prayer, Scripture reading, confession and absolution. In and through such functions, the pastor makes explicit, through word and ritual, the presence and love of God. The kerygma (proclamation) is clear and decisive.

Some pastoral functions are "covertly pastoral" in that they do not require the pastoral office and may indeed include the employment of skills and methods derived from nontheological disciplines. Such functions come closer to *diakonia* (loving acts) than to kerygma (verbal proclamation). In and through such covert functions, the communication of God's presence is more likely to be nonverbal, that is, communicated through the relationship and the acts themselves. Such functions could be seen as "the masks of God," representing "the unobvious communication of the Gospel."

The difference between overt and covert is in the *means of disclosure*, not necessarily in the theological assumptions, personal faith commitment, or role of the pastor. When providing either function, the pastor's identity is fully known to patients and staff. Covert functioning does not imply that the pastor goes incognito or underground.

The unique training and skills of today's hospital chaplains equip them with skills and methods to carry out their basic pastoral role in ways that go beyond the usual, customary, and traditional. And, of course, sometimes these methods are confusing and disturbing to patients who are expecting the usual, customary, and traditional. We saw this conflict between Chaplain Holman and Patient Iverson. Their impasse was not a disagreement over pastoral role, but rather over pastoral functions.

Many hospital chaplains today function as group therapy leaders, alcoholism counselors, crisis interveners, marriage therapists, program coordinators, psychotherapists. These functions do not in themselves require the pastoral office. In fact, these functions are performed by many professionally trained people (e.g., social workers, psychologists, nurses, psychiatrists, physicians). In performing such common functions, these professionals dip into a common pool of knowledge and theories and methods. On the surface there may be little to differentiate these professionals in the performance of these shared functions.

This is not to suggest that each will perform these functions, these shared clinical tasks, in an identical manner. They won't. Their own particular discipline will influence how each perceives and performs the functions (certainly, a theological perspective will influence how a pastor assumes these functions). The point is that these are *shared* functions, and do not in themselves require the uniqueness of the pastoral office. Through such functions, however, the pastoral role can be covertly expressed.

Often, of course, the overt and the covert blend together. Often one leads to the other. For instance, what begins as "an overt pastoral function"—a request to bring the sacrament of Holy Communion—may turn into a counseling relationship, with a sharp focus upon the dynamics and needs being expressed in that behavior the patient now considers sinful. Or, what begins as "a covert pastoral function"—a nurse's request to assess a patient's bizarre, suspicious thinking—may lead to the acknowledgment of guilt for a past transgression and a desire for confession and absolution.

This is not to suggest, however, that an appeal for one type of function always camouflages the need for another type. Sometimes a patient wants only to pray and nothing more. Sometimes a patient wants only to vent rage and nothing more. We cannot, and must not, assume that every request for prayer suggests some deeper psychological disturbance; or that every expression of anger suggests some deeper religious yearning.

It is best, of course, to respond to needs as they are expressed and to allow the relationship initiated by those needs to find its own character and depth.

Some may find such distinctions between role and function, overt and covert, arbitrary and strained. I offer them as sources of help in defining, maintaining, and (if need be) defending a pastoral identity in the multidisciplined, multifunctioning, pluralistic setting of the hospital.

A Rationale for Many Functions

One might suggest that chaplains have confused matters by engaging in a variety of functions, many of which are covert. This may be true, but there are compelling reasons that provide a rationale for such diverse pastoral functions.

Diversity of Functions Follows Diversity of Training

The breadth of chaplaincy training has broadened the potential starting points for initiating ministry. New skills uncover new needs which in turn provide new clinical entries.

Such diversity of skills and functions has enabled the chaplain to be a more integral part of "the healing community." When chaplains remain exclusively in overt, "set-apart," pastoral functions, they tend to be just that: exclusive and set apart. While this provides independence, it also breeds professional isolation. Sharing similar skills, language, and functions with other professionals usually results in peer inclusion and peer respect. Chaplains tend to find this professional comraderie stimulating and gratifying. For many, it is a new experience (many chaplains I know found their former parish ministry to be professionally isolating). Such interprofessional comraderie has also enlarged the chaplain's influence over clinical decisions and services. That influence can directly impact patient care, for where there is peer inclusion and respect, there is also "voice" and "vote" on such services.

Diversity of Functions Recognizes the Wholeness of Persons

When a pastor confines ministry to overt, set-apart functions, there is always the danger that the patient's spirituality will be seen as separate and set apart rather than as integral. Persons are a totality. Religious faith impacts and is impacted by all facets of life. Responding to a variety of needs through a multitude of functions offers the chaplain a vivid reminder of "the ecology" of persons.

Daniel Day Williams spoke convincingly of "the principle of linkage."[3] By that he meant that every part of one's life experience is linked with every other part. In other words, there is no happening in life that does not affect the whole person. A trivial incident may lead to an ultimate discovery; a light illness may be the occasion to recognize one's finite powers. Seemingly meaningless events may be the occasions to go to the roots of one's being. Immediate practical problems may be the doors through which we walk into the arena where ultimate questions are asked and answered.

Needs link to other needs. "How can I save my marriage?" may yield yet another question, "How can God's love be a part of our marital love?"

Awareness is progressive. "What does God want me to do on this matter?" may yield yet another question, "How can I be more autonomous in my decision making?"

"The principle of linkage" makes almost any starting point in a pastoral relationship a valid one, without the need to manipulate that initial concern, that presenting issue, into a religious one.

Diversity of functions recognizes that any starting point is a legitimate one; that every issue, every human concern, has a religious or spiritual dimension; and that no religious or spiritual issue is ever only that.

Diversity of Functions Recognizes the Diverse Ways in Which God's Love Can Be Communicated

God is not captive to our religious language and rituals. He is certainly no less operative when his name is not invoked, or the pastoral act is not conspicuously religious. The distinction between overt and covert pastoral functions has less to do with the reality of God than it has to do with our communication of that reality.

In overt pastoral functions, the pastor draws upon that divine power and calls attention to it. In covert pastoral functions, the pastor draws upon that same power without calling attention to it. But God's power is operative in both functions.

It would seem that the key is to have a theology of pastoral care, as well as a personal competence and confidence, that allows the needs of another to determine one's functional pastoral response. Clearly, there are those for whom the most effective ministry would be overt, a caring ministry that makes God's presence and love explicit, verbal, and clear. There are others for whom the most effective ministry would be covert, a caring ministry offered in the spirit of God's love, but without calling attention to, or making explicit reference to, the source of that love.

In both functions, the pastoral role remains unaltered, but the means by which that role is carried out varies according to the needs of people and the setting in which those personal needs are found.

Dangers in Diverse Functioning

Clearly, there are both benefits and dangers to multifunctioning. In order to be balanced in one's pastoral care it is important that one balance those benefits and dangers.

The Danger of Syncretism

In the sense used here syncretism is not a blending of religious ideologies, but a fusion of theology with the behavioral sciences. Many so-called covert functions require the employment of skills and methods (e.g., psychotherapy, crisis intervention, marriage counseling) that derive from secular sources, many of whose basic assumptions and world views are at variance with theology. A pastor who is trained to employ such skills and methods must be able and willing to acknowledge such conflicts, both potential and real. The theologically trained hospital chaplain has views of God, of human nature, sin, salvation, sanctification, eschatology, and the Holy Spirit that may be at sharp variance with these secular skills and methods. The recognition of such theoretical and practical tensions does not preclude a creative and useful integration of theology and the behavioral sciences, but should guard against a too easy accommodation of them.

The Danger of Imbalance

Shared clinical functions, professional peer inclusion, can be so satisfying that they totally consume the chaplain's interests and energies. When this occurs, covert functions predominate and overt functions are neglected, thereby making it difficult to distinguish a chaplain's identity from that of other clinicians. Paul Pruyser warns that in a multidisciplinary team there is always the danger of "levelling," in which one's pastoral functioning is indistinguishable from that of other professionals' functioning.[4] Carried to the extreme, excessive levelling means everybody adopts basically the same orientation. In such instances, Pruyser cautions, the most powerful profession predominates, usually psychiatry in psychiatric units. (In the general hospital it would be medicine.)

While Pruyser is addressing the context of a psychiatric hospital, much that he says can be applied, in principle, to a general hospital. He calls for a "sharpening," whereby each discipline "creates its own data, develops its own language."[5] This is essential because human suffering is so multifaceted and mysterious that it cannot be reduced to a single system of explanation. Sufferers need to voice their anguish in any ways they can. The multiplicity of professions, with their multiplicity of "languages," provides a multitude of opportunities for patients to voice their suffering.

What Pruyser calls for is "a perspectival approach," whereby each discipline on the treatment team can potentially address a variety of needs, but in its own way—with its own background, conceptual systems, basic premises, aims, and operational procedures.[6] I do not interpret Pruyser to mean that a pastor should be confined to overt pastoral functions. Rather, he points to the dangers of consistently subsuming that unique pastoral role in a variety of shared clinical functions.

Today's Challenge

To effect and maintain a balance in pastoral functions—to validate both the overt and covert—is the compelling challenge that confronts today's hospital chaplain. This means that the chaplain be free and able:

> to proclaim God's word clearly and decisively when the occasion calls for it, without assuming that God is captive to that word or that his presence cannot be communicated or experienced in any other way than through kerygma;

> to employ clinical skills and methods that come from nontheological sources, when the occasion calls for them, without losing sight of God's participation in them whether or not that involvement is acknowledged by deliverer and/or recipient.

When this freedom and balance are maintained, a chaplain can remain faithful to a basic pastoral role (to help others experience as fully as possible the reality of God's presence and love) and yet fulfill that role in a variety of creative and relevant ways. For indeed, a hospital chaplain has one primary role which can be and is carried out through many functions.

NOTES

1. Paul Tillich, "The Theology of Pastoral Care," *Pastoral Psychology* 10, no. 97 (October 1959): 22.

2. For a fuller discussion of this theme, see Thomas Oden, *Kergyma and Counseling* (Philadelphia: Westminster Press, 1966), chapters 1 and 2, pp. 15–83.

3. Daniel Day Williams, *Minister and the Care of Souls* (New York: Harper & Row, 1961), p. 26–27.

4. Paul Pruyser, "Religion in the Psychiatric Hospital—A Reassessment," *Journal of Pastoral Care* 38 no. 1 (March 1984): 6.

5. Ibid., p. 7.

6. Ibid., p. 6.

·PART II·

THE HOSPITAL CHAPLAIN:
Listening to the
Voices of Suffering

5
Hospitalization: A Rite of Passage

JOHN KATONAH

Without question, temporary confinement in a hospital is a pivotal point in one's life. What emerges from that experience will vary: for some it is a time of personal transformation and growth, for others it is a stultifying period marked by rhetorical questioning and bitter resentment.

What makes the difference? Where, if at all, is the sense of sacred found within the walls of suffering and pain? How can pastoral care facilitate growth and transformation in the process? Is there a way of conceptualizing the hospital experience that might be helpful both to the patient and the pastor?

In many ways traditional pastoral care, with its major emphasis upon a sacramental ministry, has unintentionally missed its mark in enabling and facilitating spiritual growth through this period of upheaval. Part of its failure has been its inadvertent tendency to limit or narrow the spiritual to the sacramental. However, the sense of the sacred is much broader, more profound, and more expansive.

What is being proposed in this chapter is a concept to help us better understand the process of hospitalization and in so doing facilitate more effective pastoral care. That concept is "rite of passage," with a primary emphasis upon "initiation." Initiation is the traditional way cultures have sought to define and describe personal crises of meaning. It embodies our whole being: mind, emotion, body, spirit, relationships. It is a sacred process, a journey from the familiar and the secure into the unfamiliar and unknown, resulting in personal change and new visions and directions for the future.

It is my contention that the concept of initiation may be a helpful means of understanding the crisis of hospitalization. It may also be a means of bringing suffering and salvation into creative dialogue and of enabling the hospitalized patient to assume a more self-conscious, participatory role in the healing process.

This chapter will attempt to refine and further develop the concept of initiation by (1) defining its three major phases; (2) relating it to hospitalization; (3) identifying its implications for hospital chaplaincy.

Three Stages of Initiation

Initiations, or rites of passage, have been studied with great curiosity by anthropologists who have traveled to numerous cultures to observe, photograph, tape record, and otherwise document these ceremonies. The reason for all of the travel, anthropologists explain, is to identify cultures uncomplicated by technological and bureaucratic smoke screens. They claim that studying initiation rites in a primitive society presents a simplified manifestation of what is entailed in this transformation process. And, as the argument continues, once "a purer form of initiation" can be pieced together from comparative studies of many primitive cultures, we can then begin to look at this process of initiation from within our own Western culture.[1]

After years of such study and documentation, there has emerged a predominant process which occurs throughout these rites of passage, even though they may take different forms and shapes and follow divergent story lines (myths).

The process of initiation breaks down into three phases: *separation, betwixt and between,* and *transformation.*

Separation

The first phase can be identified as separation.[2] The individual at puberty leaves home, family, friends, and those persons and belongings which are familiar. In male initiations, the individual leaves his village and is taken, often away from his mother, to a place outside of his usual stamping grounds. In the female's initiation, the individual is usually not taken so far away but is left to remain separated for a designated period of time. In both cases, a separation begins this ceremony. It is a time when the initiate, through societal norms and customs, consents to prepare oneself for a very real and significant transformation, while submitting to an assortment of events and happenings, according to the culture's customs. In consenting in this manner, the individual enters a foreign world. The shift from the familiar to this foreign situation is always remarkable — frequently associated with unusual costume, purification rites, music, and a change in environment. A quickened sense of life's fragility is experienced as the initiate enters this first phase of the initiation. It is a time of submission and complete trust as one turns one's life over to the customs of the village *and* to the forces within the universe.

Betwixt and Between

The second phase of initiation is one of being betwixt and between.[3] The individual is neither defined by one's old identity/roles/status nor by any newly forged identity. Nonentity would be the most accurate word for defining the person's status during this phase. Hence, all responsibilities and tasks are relinquished and the person is freed up to become totally absorbed in the initiation.

The individual's birth name is often removed to await a new name which will emerge at the conclusion of the initiation.[4] This betwixt-and-between phase describes that sense of being lost, with no familiar landmarks to help determine one's way. The initiate encounters tests of strength, endurance, wisdom, courage, and faith. These tests require responses which summon all of one's inner resources.

This phase of transition marks the time when a personal encounter with a deity may occur. Through this encounter one recognizes that one is not in total control of life but is submissive to a larger force at work. The initiate engages this deity through a ritualistic acting out of "the culture's mythic story."[5] This mythic story becomes the crucial dimension to the second phase of initiation.

The mythic story is found in all initiations. The story varies from one culture to another, but the significance always lies in the belief that it is inherently sacred and holy. The story reflects the deity's values and purposes, which in turn reflects the community's values. The reenactment of the story (which requires community participation) lifts the participants outside of time so that the story is miraculously experienced as if it is occurring for the first time.

So this mythic story then embodies a twofold purpose for the community as well as the initiate: it is an embodiment of the origin, meaning, and purpose of the culture as established by the deity; and it is also the mutually supportive avenue by which secular and sacred leave the realm of time and become reunited in the present.

The mythic story is based on a historical event that, through legend and folklore, has been passed down through the ages to the present time. It explains the role of each participant within the initiation and also provides meaning and substance to the rituals. But inevitably the story gives a transforming sense of courage and power to the participant, for it is the initiate who is enacting a sacred journey previously traveled by many initiates. These characters in the mythic story are not just acting —they *become* the lion, the demons, the arrow, the wind, the goddess, the sun.[6]

As the second phase of initiation completes its course, the initiate is brought together with the elders, or guides, of the community to begin a new identity which will have bonding with them.

If this is a male initiation rite, the boy will begin to associate (i.e., sit with, smoke with, eat with) with the older men in the community. If this is a female initiation rite, the girl becomes surrounded by adult women who clothe her in adult costumes which clearly symbolize the emergence of a new, more mature person. A clearer sense of the initiate's identity and future begins to take shape.

Transformation

The final phase is one of transformation.[7] What was emerging in the betwixt-and-between phase continues with mounting *clarity* and new *vision*. Clarity is experienced through identification with the elders of the community and through new roles and responsibilities that coincide with a new sense of accomplishment, maturation, and inner achievement. It is the new vision, with its purpose and mission, that brings the individual to a communally recognized status and role within the community. The initiate has come face to face with personal death as well as the death of an old identity. Also the initiate has experienced the deity and has thereby been touched by the sacred. It is through such experiences that the individual is considered changed and transformed. The community acknowledges that transformation by conferring upon the individual new responsibilities and a new set of costumes. These acknowledge that new strength and maturity have emerged from this initiation. The initiate is given a new name to confirm that new identity.

Various media are used to characterize this transformation: the music may drastically change in tempo and/or pathos; the initiate is clothed in celebrative, bright garments; in some societies, a new home is constructed by the community and presented as a gift. New roles are immediately ascribed thereby providing an immediate access to status and acceptance.

Anthropologists have spoken to the participants of these initiations and heard described a sense of the sacred. The initiate is encouraged to review the past events of the initiation and to reflect upon their personal meaning. This reflection is usually done with one's "new" peers, who aid in the interpretive process. Given that initiation rites are viewed as sacred, it is understandable that participants experience a sense of awe and wonder. The transformation is both *outward* (via already described physical alterations) and *inward* (through a maturation process that includes increased societal roles and a heightened sense of one's calling and mission).

Hospitalization as a Rite of Initiation

In American society hospitalization may provide a structure for initiation. Or, more to the point, I think we have already created a possibility for an initiation process. Consider this process through the example of an individual I shall call George.

George begins to be aware of physical or mental discomfort and, after attempting to use the old remedies and suggestions that others have recommended, he finally decides to make an appointment with his physician. Upon careful examination, George is admitted to the hospital. This decision to enter the hospital is not an easy one for George because it means temporarily relinquishing control over his life. He will be placing himself in the hands of others; separating himself from his neighborhood, vocation, faith community, family, and many other aspects of his life that are familiar and routine. Upon admission, he must answer many personal questions about his finances, job, habits, and relationships. Once in his room, George sheds his clothes and is given a hospital gown to wear. He is encouraged to send all jewelry and other valuables home with relatives. A name tag, with an identification number and doctor's name, is securely taped to his wrist. And the waiting begins.

Family members and friends are restricted on the time and number of visits. Hospital schedules and routines are imposed, freedom is restricted. Institutional living replaces a personal life-style. Roommate selection, noise level, accessibility to fresh air, food choices, physician and nurse visits, mobility in and out of bed, are not within George's control. Separation from the norm is dramatically experienced. This first phase, *separation,* begins the initiation process. George has left his familiar and established world for one which appears, upon first impressions, like an alien planet.

If George is able to accept the need for such a separation, he can then prepare himself for what is the *betwixt-and-between* phase of initiation: the lab tests, examinations, diagnostic work-ups, scans, cultures, X rays, and consultations. George is a courageous man and tries to portray an air of confidence and calmness with all that is happening to him. However, underneath this exterior, he feels a growing turmoil and anxiety. With each procedure, George becomes nervous over the level of intrusiveness which each test may induce and he worries over his ability to endure the procedure. Given the uncertainty of his future, which hangs in the balance with each test examination, the ultimate questions he is raising (spoken or unspoken) concern the longevity and goodness of his life and threatening death. Many questions get asked with little feeling of relief.

The CAT scan is planned for George. While he is maneuvered into the scanner, he feels so helpless and alone. Just being confronted by the massiveness of computerized machinery conjures up for George images of smallness. He experiences a greater sense of the interconnectedness of life but without his usual thoughts of omnipotence and control. Instead, he grasps a glimpse of participating in the ebb and flow of life. "I guess there are many others in this place who also are going through these procedures as well as I. I am no different than anyone else."

He finds himself reflecting on his life, recalling memories both warm and reassuring, as well as painful and guilt-ridden. What George has taken so much for granted, he now craves for and promises himself that once out of the hospital he will appreciate the simpler experiences of life. Rehearsing life and its lessons is what occupies George as he waits.

Supportive persons in George's life play an important role in this phase. Their very presence serves as a strong bond with life that exists outside of the hospital. Their supportive presence also communicates to George the value that is being connected to his personal world.

A host of varying professionals approaches him to discuss various facets in his life-style that need to be reviewed, modified, eliminated, strengthened. Nutritionist, social worker, financial counselor, occupational therapist, physical therapist, specialty instructors — each providing information and counsel to help prepare George for his eventual discharge from the hospital. However, with all the input being presented, George may only retain a portion of it, but he gains a clearer awareness of several values: life is precious and finite; each of us ultimately is responsible for the care of our bodies, minds, emotions, and souls; there are resources available to us when/if we need help.

George had a good upbringing in a church which his parents still attend. However, he has not found church-going a priority in recent years. His nonattendance does not preclude a developing faith, and it is during this betwixt-and-between time that George raises some basic faith issues. He searches for God's presence during this time when no one seems to fully understand what he is experiencing. Sometimes he even considers God as acting punitively, causing the pain and misery. Searching for meaning becomes a preoccupation. As his hospital stay extends beyond his expectation, his quest for meaning heightens.

During the treatment process, George begins making plans to return to his family, his community, his job. Anticipation mounts. But he also finds himself worrying about whether his symptoms will recur once discharged from the hospital. "Will I be able to function as usual? Have I lost something here which I will not be able to regain? Am I different in some way from when I first came in?"

In some way, George is groping for understanding. Somehow, the recent experience has aroused his curiosity and his anxiety. To simply minimize this anxious anticipation in George is to do him a disservice. It is to fail to recognize a transforming quality that has taken place during his hospitalization. George has been separated from his secure and familiar world. He has been through the wilderness of tests and procedures; he has felt the unknown in the betwixt-and-between moments. Now he is being prepared to return to the old world. But George will be entering it with new insights into his life. That changes everything.

George removes his hospital gown and shoes and replaces them with his own street clothes. His wrist band is removed, and his valuables returned to him. Suddenly he is not a patient anymore. The transforming phase is yet to be actualized. It cannot take place in the hospital; it must occur out in George's old world. However, a transformation has already been brewing within George, part of which may be outside his awareness. He has endured the separation and the betwixt-and-between times. He has weathered the storm and is wiser; in many ways, stronger for it. We say farewell to George as he leaves the hospital with his wife and daughter. Whatever happens in George's life, he can feel confident that he has been through an important initiation.

Implications for Pastoral Care

What implications does this perspective on hospitalization as a rite of initiation bring to pastoral care? One central and descriptive image for me is the image of a maieutic helper.[8] The term *maieutic* refers to the art of midwifery: that person who, during pregnancy and labor, guides and encourages the woman through the transition period to birth.

The term *maieutic* is defined by *Webster's New Twentieth Century*

Dictionary as "designating the Socratic method of helping a person to bring forth and become aware of his latent ideas or memories." In *Thaetetus* Plato depicts Socrates as one who encounters people in philosophical dialogue. Socrates describes himself as inheriting his mother's skill in midwifery by bringing to birth the mental concepts of those whose souls are pregnant with ideas. "And the greatest thing in my art is this: to be able to test, by every means, whether it's an imitation and a falsehood that the man's intellect is giving birth to, or something genuine and true."[9]

This is akin to the chaplain's role within the context of initiation. Unless one is encouraged and guided, there is the danger that the initiate will become engulfed by the chaos of hospitalization.

As the midwife needs to be present during the journey of labor, delivery, and initial care of the infant, so the chaplain is needed to affirm the patient's "journeying." This is particularly crucial during the betwixt-and-between phase of initiation. For it is in this phase that the patient perceives the experience as inactivity, not as progress or journeying.

To be in the betwixt and between phase is to travel like a nomad. It is common to feel stuck because the journey seems aimless and endless. However, if the maieutic helper affirms and redefines the feeling of inactivity as part of a sacred journey experience, then an openness to the sacred and the possibility for an initiation process may begin. This can be done as the patient is helped to elucidate personal experiences during this phase, whether through the use of traditional and religious words or images (e.g., "wandering through the wilderness like the Hebrews in the desert") or through personal associations with past memories (e.g., "that CAT scan reminded me of the time I delivered my first child"). By identifying unique, idiosyncratic symbols and images that are expressed, the maieutic helper can affirm the journey. By encouraging a significant story or myth that grows out of the individual's hospitalization experience, the chaplain can help the patient to redefine the significance of his or her hospitalization.

One patient I encountered was a vibrant, active woman of twenty-five who had been stricken with multiple sclerosis since the age of seventeen. She had been in and out of hospitals since that time for one treatment or surgery after another. When I met her she was having difficulty with urinary retention. After contracting multiple sclerosis, this young woman had gone on to finish high school, attended and completed paramedic training, and was in the process of applying to medical school in hopes of becoming a physician. Although she never graphically described the "story" of her experience through her illness, she periodically did share some of her beliefs which aided her journey. She spoke of her body as if it were separate from the rest of her, yet conversed about it (her body) as if talking about an old, dear friend. At times she could laugh at her uncooperative arms or legs. I once walked into her room and found her scolding her arm for not contributing its part in making her lunch time pleasurable. In her ability to separate from, yet remain connected to, her ailing body, this woman then was able to embrace life and make plans to accomplish certain goals and dreams which she set before herself. And when a setback occurred (like returning to the hospital), she naturally felt some sadness and regret but eventually revamped her plans and soon was involved in new ways of remaining creative: reading, pen sketching, attempting to remain independent and self-sufficient.

From such stories, which each of us creates or draws upon in life's transitional crossroads, can emerge personal meaning in our experiences of pain and loss. Through such a story, the patient finds a way of participating in the event of hospitalization, rather than being a helpless, passive victim.

In the separation phase, patients frequently experience an inability to accept their own finiteness. This is accompanied by a lack of trust of others. If one does not appreciate one's own limitations and weaknesses, then surely one will have little understanding or acceptance of one's dependency. Therefore, one cannot trust the helpful efforts of others. As a maieutic helper, the chaplain can attempt to bring a trusting presence to the relationship, which in turn might facilitate the patient's confrontation with fear and helplessness. By supporting the patient's very decision to enter the hospital, the chaplain can help to foster the recognition that there are times in life when we need and must call upon others for help.

Speaking to an elderly man hospitalized for a bruised rib cage and pneumonia, I discovered that his wife suddenly had taken ill a year prior, and shortly thereafter died. This man still could not understand how she could die before him since he was so much older and sicker than she. He described how much he savored reading historical and political writings except during the very late evening hours when, because of his inability to sleep, he found himself drawn to reading mystery novels, sometimes not putting them down until he completed the whole novel. I interpret this repeated occurrence as symbolizing this man's repetitious search for resolution of the mystery, and the mystery continues to be: "Why did my wife die?" This individual was stuck in the separation phase and struggling to find his way through the "mystery."

In the betwixt-and-between phase, one can clearly appreciate issues of faith and justice during those moments when the usual familiar landmarks for assessing the value of life are missing. During such times one often sinks into self-debasement and self-recrimination. Confession may be an important part of this phase. But unless it is balanced by the assurance of God's forgiveness, the betwixt-and-between phase can feel like an eternal hell.

Also manifest within this phase of initiation is the sense of the holy. As a maieutic helper, the chaplain can be a strong, positive force in affirming the patient's own belief in that sense of the holy. This can often be done by relating the biblical image of journeying as it relates to the patient's own current experience. Or the chaplain may also refer to personal, nontraditional experiences to nourish the idea of journeying. The chaplain must endure and accept the tremendous anxiety felt and acted out by patients during this difficult betwixt-and-between phase.

Diagnosed with breast cancer two years earlier, a woman entered the hospital because of lower-back pain. Her physicians quickly ascertained that she had bone cancer and were concerned that she evaded any discussions about her disease. Pastoral care was called. In our short visit she hesitatingly shared an image which was both confusing and frightening. She described seeing herself seated in a rocking chair, calmly rocking. At a distance she began noticing something approaching. As it got closer, she could not make out the form or content. Once within close range, she began to push the "thing" away with her hands. Her efforts to do so were in vain. She continued to be confused about what this object was and why it was encroaching upon her. This scenario was repeated over and over. She perceived the "thing" as destructive and judgmental of her past. She also spoke of feeling alienated from others because she could not determine how or with whom to share this. More importantly, however, the patient described much relief in now sharing it and being assured that her vision might contain a helpful message. Being able to accept this experience as potentially healing rather than destroying became a redeeming insight for her.

The third phase of initiation (transformation) is one not usually experienced in the hospital. However, for those who do express a sense of transformation, spiritual issues which emerge focus around gratefulness (grace) that one is now able to experience. The patient often confronts some important questions. Can one identify signs of transformation and change? Can one resolve grief over the loss of the old and begin to affirm the new?

Another spiritual issue in this phase is the sense of vocation and communion with life. This refers to "a person's willingness to be a cheerful participant in the scheme of creation and providence, so that a sense of purpose is attached to one's doings which validates his existence under his Creator." [10] This sense of purpose then can be viewed as having emerged from one's encounter with the sacred through the experience. Frequently these transforming signs and purposes are not clearly evident. Indeed, contemplation and reflection are needed in order to assimilate the intensity of the initiation and to get in touch with physical, social, emotional, spiritual changes that have occurred.

As a maieutic helper, the chaplain blesses the initiation and reaffirms it as a sacred journey. Ritual may be appropriate during this transforming time, since ritual can provide structure for reflecting on these recent events. Inclusion of family and friends in this rite will also affirm the individual as a member of the community and welcome that person back into society.

An example of someone whose spiritual issue centered around a sense of purpose comes to mind. A woman many years earlier had one of her kidneys removed. Over the past three years she had been battling cancer cells which had invaded her colon. With each stage of cancer, her doctors made recommendations and she would consent. But she never experienced any freedom. "Either I do what they say or I die. That's not much of a choice." During her last hospitalization her remaining kidney became dysfunctional. After several weeks of being on dialysis (kidney machine), her doctors again came to her with their recommendations and her "options." Her decision was to discontinue dialysis and return home to her husband. When I visited her in her home, she stated that her decision to stop medical treatment was a profound relief. She admitted that it was the first time in the past three years that she had made a decision that was totally her own. She was thereby able to exert her control over her situation. Remarkably, as we talked further, she recounted how many friends, as well as hospital staff, had supported her in this decision and openly admired her courage. Although she was not able to appreciate what others appeared to appreciate in her, she felt at peace with the idea that she had "left my mark on the world" through this decision. This feeling of accomplishment left her awaiting death with a sense of peace and fulfillment.

Conclusion

As the maieutic helper, the chaplain provides direction and structure to a process through the initiation model of hospitalization. Both the midwife and the chaplain utilize those resources which the "patient" brings to the transforming experience. This model of hospitalization and pastoral care has only been touched in these pages. The possibilities for aiding this transforming experience are vast, awaiting only the chaplain's imagination and creativity.

If one were to transpose these rite-of-passage concepts to practical use within a medical setting, one might find the hospital itself may be transformed. Architecturally and functionally I would envision a hospital that includes windows that open and allow influx of fresh air when desired. Terraces on each floor would be accessible to patients and family members for the healing rays of the sun. Space on each unit would be provided for patients to congregate and to share their experiences with other "initiates." There also would be a policy, respected by all hospital staff, which granted patients thirty minutes of uninterrupted quiet each day in which to read, contemplate, pray, meditate, or to do anything else that appealed to their interest. An abundance of plant life would be growing throughout the hospital. All commercial TV would be eliminated and FM radios with headphones would be installed by each patient's bed to provide a variety of listening music.

Also placed by the patient's bed, along with the traditional Bible, would be books on artwork (i.e., painting, sculpting, carving, molding, soldering) as well as works of poetry, short stories, fairy tales, folklore. Plays, concerts, and dramatic readings would be regularly offered in the hospital auditorium for patients, families, and staff. A greater variety of artwork would be displayed throughout the hospital as well as within patients' rooms. These paintings would reflect scenes and settings which span human emotions. There would even be innovative crafts available to patients to facilitate various media for them to express their journey of hospitalization. Needless to say, all of these innovations would be enacted as ways of stimulating one's total senses, as well as calling forth one's creative energy, toward identifying a personal "mythic story."

Hospitalization is a time of separation and turmoil and mystery. It can, however, be a time of sacred journeying—leaving us, upon discharge, prepared to embrace life anew, with new skills and strengths that we have come to discover. Pastoral care needs to play a role in this journey so that more individuals may experience the creative possibility of new life through this rite of initiation known as hospitalization.

NOTES

1. Victor Turner, *Ritual Process: Structure and Anti-Structure* (New York: Cornell Paperbacks: Cornell University Press, 1969), p. v.

2. Arnold Van Gennep, *Rites of Passage*, trans. M. Vizedom and G. Caffee (London: Routledge and Kegan Paul, 1909), p. 10ff.

3. Ibid.

4. Bruce Lincoln, *Emerging From the Chrysalis* (Cambridge: Harvard University Press, 1981), p. 79.

5. Ibid., p. 95.

6. Steven Foster and Meredith Little, *Book of the Vision Quest* (California: Island Press, 1980), p. 91.

7. Van Gennep, *Rites of Passage*, p.10ff.

8. Lecture by Janet Stein, Ph.D, at the C.C. Jung Center, Evanston, Illinois, on "Initiation and Archetypes" (October 1982).

9. Plato, *Thaetetus*, trans. with notes by John McDowell (London: Clarendon Press Oxford, 1973), p. 13.

10. Paul Pruyser, *Minister as Diagnostician* (Philadelphia: Westminster Press, 1976), p. 76.

6

The Random Initial Visit

LAWRENCE E. HOLST

A unique characteristic of hospital chaplaincy is "the right" of initiative. By that is meant the chaplain's license to intervene without the special sanctions of a referral or a patient's request. As someone once described it: "The chaplain needs no passport to enter any patient's room." Such geographic initiative provides the hospital chaplain broad access to all patients.

Granted, the chaplain is not the only member of the hospital community who makes unannounced, unscheduled visits. A nurse will stop in to take temperatures, a lab technician to draw blood, a medical resident to take a history, a nutritionist to discuss diets. These people, too, will be strangers to the patient. Unlike the chaplain, however, they come under the broad spectrum of medical authority to execute medical orders. They are part of "the hospital routine." Their presence and services are expected.

What distinguishes the chaplain's random initial visits is not anonymity (other hospital personnel are equally unknown) or their unexpectedness (other hospital personnel stop in unexpectedly). Rather, it is the unknown relationship of the chaplain's visits to medical care and the unforeseen images that such a presence stimulates.

The right of geographic initiative is a valuable vestige of pastoral care's rich heritage. It is "a custom of the discipline." It is essentially the *chaplain's freedom to create and control the time, place, setting in which, and persons to whom, pastoral care is to be offered.*

The right of initiative brings together many unique dimensions of pastoral care, namely, mobility, freedom of access, and control over the expenditure of time and skills. Obviously, such rights of initiative do not preclude pastoral responsiveness to others' initiatives. They simply open up another pastoral option.

The warrants for such initiative are varied. In the parish, such warrants are bequeathed through the covenant struck between pastor and congregation in the rite of installation. In the hospital, such warrants generally come through administrative or board decree. However, the sanctions are deeper even than those. *They are inherent in the office of ministry.* Clergy are expected to intersect people in crisis. Indeed, more likely it is not their presence, but their absence that draws criticism. Clergy are part of a vast supportive network available to those in need. That supportive role does not have to be earned; it is conferred by both the church and society.

The random initial hospital visit is but one expression of that conferred right. Yet despite its broad endorsement, it is a difficult type of ministry. It demands diligence, persistence, flexibility, spontaneity, and patience. At times, the initiating hospital chaplain feels like a traveling salesman. Like salesmanship, initial visits require aggressiveness. They risk rejection. At best, the initiating chaplain is uninvited; at worst, the chaplain is unwelcomed.

Consider the differences when the chaplain is requested to make a visit by a patient. Then the chaplain is a *responder*, rather than an *initiator* and can assume that this patient:

has a recognized need for which one is now seeking pastoral help;

has a sense of personal responsibility for that need, or at least owns the responsibility to do something about it;

has a motivation to act upon that need now;

has a willingness to entrust that need to an as yet unknown, unseen hospital chaplain.

Of course, these factors do not assure a favorable therapeutic outcome. But they do clarify the respective roles of initiator and responder. The responding chaplain has every right to assume that the initiating patient will define a reason for the requested visit.

However, when the chaplain initiates a visit the roles are reversed. The chaplain cannot presume needs, motivation, trust, or readiness in the patient. Nor can the chaplain presume that the patient will bear any responsibility for the visit, or even elect to utilize the services that are being offered. In a random initial visit the chaplain has chosen the patient for ministry; the patient has not yet chosen the chaplain to minister. In fact, that choice may never be made.

Though these factors seem less favorable, this is not to suggest that a very strong, productive relationship cannot be established under such conditions. The point is that the initiator of the relationship bears initial responsibility for its definition and direction. If such a relationship continues, then that responsibility will become mutual.

In a random initial visit the controls are evenly distributed. The initiating chaplain controls the time and place of the visit. The chaplain also enters the relationship with some vital information about the patient: name, age, address, religion, next of kin, physician's name, admitting diagnosis, estimated length of stay. Indeed, the chaplain may know some factors about the patient that the patient doesn't know. And, of course, the patient knows nothing about the chaplain at this point in the relationship. Neither patient nor chaplain "controls" the environment. Interruptions, phone calls, visitors, examinations, monitorings may occur without notice.

However, as responder, the patient retains considerable control and can accept or reject the chaplain's initiative. Rejections can be direct ("chaplain, I'm really not interested") or indirect (by indifference and avoidance). The chaplain cannot compel the patient to participate; without such participation it is difficult to foresee a meaningful interaction.

The initiating chaplain cannot presume the right to focus upon the patient's needs, even if discerned. While a broad license has been accorded a chaplain's physical initiative, no such license has been given for "psychological intrusion." Such license can only be given by the patient. So, in a deeper sense, a chaplain's initiative does not violate a patient's autonomy.

In fact, strange though it may seem, the relationship between the initiating chaplain and the responding patient is quite symmetrical, characterized by considerable mutuality and equality. Neither is in a superior position. Both can remain disengaged. Either can drop or pursue the relationship.

If the two of them do pursue further visits, the relationship may become structured and focused. On the other hand, future visits may remain unstructured, diffused, and scattered. The potential outcomes resulting from a random hospital initial visit are diverse. This is true, in part, because of the hospital setting, but also because the symmetrical relationship tends to evenly divide controls and options.

Advantages and Disadvantages of Random Initial Visits

As one has already surmised, the right of pastoral initiative is a mixed blessing. There are advantages:

Initiative allows the pastor to reach people in their earliest stages of need. Crises often immobilize even the quest for help. The physical presence of the pastor may be all that is necessary to facilitate that quest. Studies in crisis intervention stress the factor of *immediacy*: to achieve close timing between precipitating crisis events and the entry of help. If intervention is early, disequilibrium can be more healthily resolved before maladaptive coping resources become crystallized. The early entry of help also takes advantage of heightened energy stimulated in the early phases of a crisis.

Some people have needs they cannot readily articulate; some have needs that are too threatening to articulate. To seek help for such needs may be difficult and embarrassing. However, to respond to help that suddenly presents itself at their bedsides may be much easier. Initiative provides the visibility of help which often leads to its utilization.

Initiative reduces the need for a cumbersome referral process. Since pastoral care is not a required medical service, it is easy for hospital personnel to neglect its usefulness. In fact, part of pastoral care's value is its detachment from medical delivery. Many patient interactions have to do with medical concerns. When a chaplain drops by, the patient has the unusual opportunity to share matters that are not exclusively medical, yet are deeply important.

Pastoral initiative makes available services that might be missed if they were limited to staff referral or patient request. Staff may not know how to integrate such services into the medical spectrum; patients may not know such resources are available.

Since pastoral care falls outside the parameters of medical treatment, the chaplain's initiative is not perceived by staff to be intrusive or competitive with their services and, in most instances, is welcomed.

Initiative is the patient's due. The costs of pastoral care are "hidden" in most hospital budgets. Chaplains do not charge patients for visits made. Such costs are part of the patient's room rate. This makes it possible for the chaplain to take initiative and to expend lavish amounts of time on patients whose needs seem to warrant it.

Of course, if pastoral care was a fee for service, random initial visits would be presumptuous. One can imagine the consternation of patients who would be billed for pastoral visits they didn't request.

Consequently, one might maintain that every patient is entitled to an initial visit since pastoral care is part of every patient's medical costs.

As well, there are disadvantages to pastoral initiatives:

A psychological burden is always upon the initiator. Initiation carries with it the burden of defining the nature and purpose of the encounter.

One cannot expect hospitalized patients to understand the ground rules and parameters of a visit they did not request. Nor can one expect them to bear responsibility for defining and developing the relationship.

Taking initiative with strangers (which is the case in random hospital initial visits) can be very difficult, especially for chaplains who are shy and reserved. Such chaplains would much prefer responding to patients' initiative.

Initiative may get ahead of a patient's readiness and motivation. Clearly, such unscheduled visits may be upon the wrong persons, in the wrong place, at the wrong time. The patient may be drowsy, talked out, uncomfortable, in pain, or just plain grouchy. Some patients may say too little; others may say too much (in their unguarded vulnerability they may blurt out things they mean, but did not mean to say). For most, it takes time to feel secure in a new relationship. A brief unannounced, unscheduled visit by a stranger usually does not provide the security required for openness.

Initiative may result in many vague, undefined, diffused relationships. It is indeed difficult to have the freedom of initiative without compromising some of the "neatness" of a clearly structured, formally contracted relationship. Since the ground rules and boundaries for such surprise visits are undefined, the surprised patient may be at a loss as to how to respond. And, since the customary response to strangers is to engage in safe social chitchat, that is what random initial visits often produce. One of the hazards of pastoral initiative is that the dialogue remains at that level.

Since initiative rested with the chaplain, the patient may expect the chaplain to control the entire visit, if not the relationship. When that does not occur, and the chaplain tries to switch gears, the patient may feel confused. The resultant dialogue between them may be unfocused and rambling. As the relationship terminates, with the patient's discharge, it might be difficult for either of them to see any purpose or value to their interaction.

Initiative may foster dependency in both patients and staff. Closely related to the above is the dependency that initiative often engenders. It may be a patient's underlying assumption that the initiator begin, carry out, and terminate the visit. Passivity, acquiescence, and dependency may characterize the relationship.

Staff, too, may grow so accustomed to pastoral initiative that they fail to make referrals, assuming the chaplain will find the troubling situations, anyway. Without question, the right of initiative can easily occupy a chaplain's day, thereby reducing the need for staff referrals. As this continues, it may cause the chaplain to become more and more independent of the staff.

Guidelines for Initiative

It is not a matter of whether random initial hospital visits are more or less difficult, more or less important, than formally scheduled pastoral counseling interviews. They are different. They have their own nature and style and demand different skills.

Given that random initial visiting is a crucial, if not indispensable, ministry for the hospital chaplain, the challenge is how to maximize its potential.

The following are suggested guidelines for the random initial visit:

Define one's identity and role as clearly as possible. For starters, this means name, profession, hospital assignment, and the purpose of this introductory visit (to get acquainted). If the patients are listening and absorbing, this will at least disabuse them of two common fears about a chaplain's surprise visit: that the chaplain is from a nearby parish recruiting members; that they have been selected for this visit because of the gravity of their illness. We must never underestimate "the image of death" that chaplains bear for many.

If it seems warranted, the chaplain might provide a broad overview of one's hospital functions without giving a detailed job description.

Such an overview is important because though many patients are active members of a congregation, this may be their first, personal, one-on-one visit with a member of the clergy. The unexpected visit may be disarming. A broad description of how a chaplain spends a day in the hospital might be reassuring and also provide some clues on how the patient might utilize such services.

Ten years ago Bruce Hartung put the issue succinctly:

> The initial call will be even more difficult if the question of role expectation is allowed to remain under the table, implicit rather than explicit in the relationship. What is needed is either chaplains who are comfortable with what seem to be the overwhelming cultural expectations of what a chaplain does in the hospital (bringing Sacraments and comforting the dying) or chaplains who, in the first few minutes of an initial call, provide some kind of experience that makes explicit why the chaplain is in the room, if that "what" is different from the patient-defined role of the chaplain.[1]

Other means can be used to describe broadly a chaplain's role, such as an attractive printed brochure (distributed as part of "the admission packet," or by the chaplain in the initial visit) or a "meet the chaplain" telecast in the hospital's daily multimedia schedule.

While it is assumed that a professionally certified chaplain will have forged out a clear role definition, each chaplain is encouraged to check out that definition against the expectations of patients, staff, and hospital administration.

Without doubt, a major source of chaplain frustration is the disparity between *self's* and *others'* expectations. What is needed is a means of identifying that disparity and a willingness to seek to narrow it. As was indicated in chapter 4 above, pastoral role is determined by external and internal forces. What is needed, ultimately, is a creative blend of the two. A chaplain who submits totally to external expectations will "burn out." If a chaplain pursues only his or her internal expectations, the job may "burn out."

Be attentive to patients' reactions to your pastoral presence. It has been said that first impressions are important and lasting. That may be. However, in this regard first impressions are important clues to what the chaplain symbolizes to the patient. Initially, patients will more likely respond out of their internal images and references (provoked by the chaplain) than to external realities of the chaplain's appearance, personality, and style.

Of all the helping professions, clergy has the longest history. It is a profession that is many centuries old. Consequently, time has allowed many images, concepts, and role expectations to emerge. These have been passed on from generation to generation. Carl Jung referred to these as "archetypes."

When a pastoral relationship is initiated, many of these historic, and often unconscious, images are stimulated. Psychoanalysis has provided a concept that is helpful in describing this phenomenon. It is called *transference.* Transference is an "as if" reaction. "As if" the therapist, or counselor, or authority (in this case, chaplain) were an emotionally important person from early in one's life. Many of these internal images are highly charged by early developmental stages (e.g., the priestly designation "father" is highly suggestive of a parental-authority figure).

In this sense, transference is a response determined principally by the inner needs and conflicts of the patient rather than by the behavior of the chaplain.

Transference usually includes three psychological phenomena:

Introjection. Qualities or characteristics learned from one's parents and/or other early authorities which are then incorporated into one's own personality.

Projection. Attributing those qualities and characteristics learned from early authorities onto current authorities, whether or not they accurately "fit" those authorities.

Displacement. Expressing those feelings onto current authorities that are intended for earlier authorities; that is, responding to the past through the present.

These transference reactions are unconscious; they may be positive or negative or, most commonly, both. Thus, a chaplain's presence at a patient's bedside may provoke a combination of trust, confidence, security, anger, guilt, fear, and dependency. As stated, these emotional reactions may have little to do with the chaplain's behavior or self-image.

All human interactions have some transference. It is part of the economy of relating to "transfer" past experiences onto the present. That way we're not always starting from scratch in every relationship. Of course, current experiences can, and do, modify those images, that's why transference lessens as the relationship continues.

In an initial pastoral visit it is important to observe these "pastoral images," and "internal references." For out of them emerge reactions and expectations. From the chaplain some patients will want reprimand or chastisement, rescue or restraint; others will want sanction and encouragement, hope and optimism. Still others will want the chaplain to change their situations or the behavior of their loved ones. To be sure, some of these expectations will derive from their immediate needs, others from their unconsciously held images. Some expectations will be appropriate and realistic; others will be magical and illusory. Some requests will be communicated as demands, others as pleas. Some of these will be congruent with the chaplain's own role concept, others will be incongruent. Failure to meet such requests may be perceived by patients as pastoral unwillingness, not as inability.

This is not an appeal for hospital chaplains to become trained in the extremely complex process of transference, but rather to be aware of its presence in all relationships, particularly in an initial visit. Since most random initial hospital visits bring together two strangers, it is natural that patients will draw upon past images to gear them up for this newly created relationship.

Nor is this an appeal for chaplains to modify their role in order to meet any and all patient demands. Rather, it is an appeal to recognize the vast array of role images and expectations a chaplain encounters, many of which are engendered by transference.

Be patient with the patient. By entering a patient's room unannounced, the chaplain has the advantage of being forewarned and forearmed. It is best not to press the advantage. A discerning chaplain may uncover many patient needs in those initial minutes. It is best not to exploit them in the early phases of the relationship, lest the patient later become defensive and resistant. Sensitive restraint should characterize the chaplain's behavior during a random initial visit. Trust and confidence can only come as time allows them to be engendered.

Attempt to facilitate a role reversal. In the random initial visit the chaplain is the initiator and the patient is the responder. Many years ago, in describing "The Pre-Counseling Possibility," Seward Hiltner spoke of attempting to convert the pastor's "geographic initiative" into the counselee's (or, in this case, patient's) "psychological initiative."[2] By "psychological initiative" is meant the active utilization of the relationship to meet one's needs. For this to occur, a role reversal must be effected.

Such role reversal is a goal of the random initial visit. This means a dynamic shift for both: the chaplain shifts from "physical initiator" to "psychological responder"; the patient shifts from physical responder to psychological initiator. When this occurs, each bears responsibility for the nature and character of the relationship. Such a reversal cannot be forced. All that the initiating chaplain can do really is to provide the time and space for it to occur. Sometimes it does, sometimes it doesn't. Sometimes it occurs partially. There are many shades of grey in the process.

Some patients can't assert a claim upon the relationship; some chaplains can't let go of their initial control. Some patients don't feel a need for a role reversal; some chaplains can't hear the needs expressed.

To effect such a role reversal, to help patients assume psychological initiative in response to the chaplain's physical initiative, requires pastoral sensitivity, patience, and skill. When it occurs, the relationship has a better potential for being mutually rewarding. When it doesn't occur, the relationship must be accepted on other terms.

Determine a follow-up. Every random initial visit should conclude with a follow-up plan. Three factors will determine that follow-up:

Needs. Expressed and perceived needs become a major criterion for follow-up. In addition to the chaplain's observations, it is advisable to check out the staff's perception of needs.

Motivation. Patient needs, however, may not always be paralleled by patient motivation. Patients may choose not to deal with recognized needs during their hospitalization, or at least not with the chaplain. Patient motivation may also vary with regard to *level* (intense or slight) and to *direction* (broad or narrow). Follow-up ministry must weigh and consider both level and direction.

Where needs and motivation are at variance, it does not mean that pastoral care should cease. It simply means that style and approach will be different. Continued visits may build trust; and motivation to deal with those needs may follow that trust.

Availability. Patients' physical and emotional availability will vary. So will chaplains'.

Some patients are available for ministry but do not want it (lack of motivation); some patients want an active ministry but aren't available for it (because of drowsiness, unconsciousness, long absences from the room, anesthesia, pain, the constant presence of visitors).

A chaplain's availability will also vary. No chaplain can possibly be to all patients what they need and want. Realistic limits must be set.

Again, it is advisable to collaborate with staff so that the hospital's collective resources (including the chaplain) can be responsibly deployed according to patient need, motivation and availability.

In considering all factors, the chaplain should determine a course of action, based on the following questions:

What information should I share with staff? What do I need to learn from them?

Do I plan to initiate a revisit? Does the patient know this? Was it agreed upon?

Do I plan to revisit only at the patient's request? Does the patient know this? Does the patient know how to contact me in the hospital?

What issues need focusing in subsequent visits?

Should you and the patient agree on those issues?

Should I contact the family?

What are the realistic possibilities and limits in this relationship?

It is advisable to encourage the patient to participate in such follow-up decisions:

Would the patient like a follow-up visit?

If so, what are the preferred times?

What issues would the patient want to pursue?

Would the patient prefer initiating a follow-up visit?

Does the patient know how to do this?

By "encouraging" the patient to participate in such questions, the chaplain is helping the patient to assert "the psychological initiative," and is thereby helping to foster "a role reversal."

It is ironic that chaplains who often protest the lack of patient autonomy in hospital routines are frequently unwilling themselves to submit their services and availability to patient determination. Control can be a vital possession for a hospital chaplain.

When a chaplain and patient begin to work out together the nature of their relationship, they will inevitably have to confront issues of control and surrender, assertiveness and dependency, freedom and mutuality. When they do this, they are drawing very close to some of the key struggles of life. When properly negotiated, the chaplain's random initial visit provides the opportunity for patients to engage those major struggles in a small but significant way. And, it may provide the opportunity for the patient to see the broader implications of such vital human struggles.

NOTES

1. Bruce Hartung, "The Initial Call," in *Toward a Creative Chaplaincy*, ed. Lawrence E. Holst and Harold P. Kurtz (Springfield, Ill.: Charles C. Thomas, 1973) p. 20.
2. Seward Hiltner, *Pastoral Counseling* (New York: Abington Press, 1949), p. 129.

7

The Voices on Obstetrics:
Participants and Partners

SUSAN JOHNSON KLINE

Pregnancy is indeed a deeply sacramental time. For months we live with signs and wonders. The reality is soon fully present . . . but veiled. Love has never been so alive in me![1]

A typical response when people hear that I work on the obstetrics unit is, "Oh, that's the happy floor. You must really enjoy your work." But, to be honest, when I first began working on maternity units, I questioned the significance of my ministry.

Yet I have discovered that ministry on obstetrics can be quite significant. Just as the entire genetic code for a human being is packed into each union of ovum and sperm, so too are the seeds of spiritual issues packed into the powerful, but short-term experience of the birth of a baby. Depending on the type of experience one brings to and takes away from the birth, spiritual beliefs are encoded which may determine the shape of one's parenting. For example, some parents feel a baby is their own creation, a "product of their conception," a "possession" for which they are to be congratulated. This logic can be used to support a privatistic approach to such decisions as abortion or the discipline of a child. Others see their baby as a gift from God, lent to them only temporarily for their care, nurture, and upbringing. Such beliefs might allow for child-rearing decisions to be made in community, and with the help of external sources of authority.

One young single mother was hospitalized in the perinatal unit for two months, awaiting the birth of her child. Her symptoms were jaundice and right-side pain, thought to be hepatitis. Her child was seen not so much as a possession or a gift, but rather as a "savior," one who would make her partner stay with her. Instead, when the baby was born, the father took the boy to his home country to be raised by his extended family. A second child, born of the same parents, was later brought to the emergency room. It was suspected that the child had been abused. The baby could not fulfill the psychological and spiritual needs of the mother.

The birth of a baby can elicit other spiritual attitudes. A child can be seen by either father or mother as a competitor for a limited quantity of love; it can be seen as a threat to a new parent's sense of competency; it can be seen as the fulfillment of a partnership, the very purpose for which a couple was married.

Spiritual Themes in Pregnancy

Within the last ten years there has been a great deal of focus among pastors, physicians, and ethicists upon the dramatic obstetrical issues: stillbirths, high-risk infants, cessation-of-treatment questions, elective and therapeutic abortions, amniocentesis and genetic counseling. And yet, there are many powerful spiritual issues occurring within the lives of those families with "normal" pregnancies.

This area provides a great challenge for chaplains. How does one engage a family whose hospital contact is only two to five days in such spiritual reflection? My answer is not composed of specific techniques, but rather focuses upon the themes I hear from parents.

Participation and Partnership versus Passivity

One theme which sets a context for ministry is a cultural one: a shift from anesthetized and isolating experiences of childbirth to alert and active participation; and a movement from seeing childbirth as involving only the woman, to that of seeing it as partnership.

The popularity of such experiences as "prepared childbirth" classes, birthing rooms, the Nilsson micro-photography of the stages of fetal development,[2] the Leboyer method of "gentle birth"[3] are indications of an increasing recognition of birth as an awesome experience, one in which parents want to participate to its fullest.

Historically, childbirth has been seen as an experience for reverence, and until about twenty years ago, pregnancy was seen as a time for remaining hidden at home. However, the reverence was sometimes experienced as isolating, alienating a woman from her community and from her body. The process of labor was considered a necessary evil, requiring as much anesthesia as possible. Today, women are experiencing a greater level of acceptance of their pregnant bodies (e.g., the advent of designer maternity clothes and bathing suits), and labor is viewed as tolerable pain that can be encountered confidently as part of a child's healthy emergence into the world.

Not only is there a sense of greater participation but also an assumption that childbirth is a drama among partners: mother and child, childbirth coach (usually father) and mother, doctor and parents. Today, women who give birth seem to be letting go of an image of motherhood as their *only* vocation, one which demands wholehearted commitment. Instead, they are viewing parenthood as partnership, expecting equal participation with their husbands in providing a home, earning financial support, and rearing the children.

Just as there has been a cultural shift toward increasing knowledge of bodily processes and increasing participation in the birthing process, so too there has been a shift in *the theology of parenthood*. This shift is from a theology which focused primarily on a masculine God who created man and woman "to be fruitful and multiply" (the woman "to have pain in childbearing") to a God with whom we are in responsible partnership as co-creators, and in whom we can recognize both masculine and feminine faces. We are partners with a God who participates in our lives from our birth to our death. By affirming the equal partnership of men and women in parenting, we can understand something of God's nature.[4]

Responsibility versus Limitations

> We intentionally prevented pregnancy for so long while we each developed our careers, I thought we were in complete control of our reproductive functions. Just stop the pill, and we'll get pregnant. It took us over a year to get pregnant, and now we've had a miscarriage. Maybe we'll never be parents.

The spiritual issues of parenthood begin with an adolescent's first awareness of sexuality and decisions about its uses. When the connection between sexuality and procreation is made, a young girl or boy is faced with the responsibility for his or her body. With the multitude of birth control methods available, one can feel some control over the decision of parenthood. Whereas the hotly debated issue in the early 1960s was whether or not to provide sex education for children in the schools, now the question has become whether to inform parents before distributing contraceptives to minors. Knowledge about sexuality is now assumed by many to be important for adolescents.

Couples are feeling greater control and, therefore, greater responsibility for their decisions to have children. Many seem to feel "conception" occurs not with the actual physical union of bodies or of ovum and sperm, but when they first "conceive" of the idea that they want children. Their concept of family leads them to plan for the arrival of children, perhaps to space children, and their prior decisions of whether and which methods of birth control to use.

We feel a godlike *responsibility*: "Be fruitful and multiply." We feel a godlike *control*: "Fill the earth and subdue it." Technology is enabling us to fulfill both responsibilities. We feel a godlike quest for *perfection*: we have new awareness of the influence of alcohol, caffeine, aspirin, exercise, hot tubs upon unborn fetuses.

In the face of all this, however, we are starkly reminded of our human limitations. Some teenagers become pregnant despite birth control; some married couples find it difficult to conceive and, despite our medical technology, some babies are born with severe physical anomalies. We feel our profound vulnerability as procreators. Even with a normal planned-for pregnancy, and a healthy delivery, we realize that our susceptibility to loss has only begun.

Yet for many, the experience of parenthood allows for the rebirth of a blissful innocence: baby clothes with ruffles, pastel comforters, and bright primary colors in the nursery all symbolize joy, new life, celebration. It is as if we are allowed to re-enter the Garden of Eden for a while. However, when something goes wrong with a pregnancy, parents are quickly confronted with the loss of their illusions and a new awareness of finitude.

Self-Realization versus Loss of Self

> The mother expecting a multiple birth had been here for two months on the perinatal unit. She was on bed rest, with bathroom privileges. Her legs and face were swollen, retaining water. Most of her day was spent in sleeping and forcing herself to eat. Her older child visited a couple of times a week. There were anxieties among the staff as to how many of the fetuses would survive. When I visited her, she spoke little of the discomforts or the anxieties, but rather smiled and said, "I'm just in the service of these little babies right now. I am content to take care of myself in hopes that they will all survive."

Arising from the sense of responsibility and vulnerability comes a question of identity. "Who am I anyway? What kind of power do I have? At times I feel a godlike power and influence over this baby; at others I feel totally in the service of this newly forming life, as if I am only a vessel." Women who have previously felt a very conditional acceptance of their bodies are called now to accept the process of growth and to make space for their child in their bodies and self-concepts. They begin to feel as if their body is no longer a private possession (during pregnancy many people feel a freedom to touch a woman's belly that they would not feel at any other time).

For some women, pregnancy and motherhood is a time of ultimate fulfillment. However, Anne Bedford Ulanov, a Jungian analyst, warns against the danger of finding one's identity solely in one's baby, thereby losing a sense of the child's otherness:

> As long as such a woman carries the unborn baby within her, the baby is felt not only as part of her body, but the best part. The baby's presence gives her identity: as a pregnant woman, entitled to courtesy, consideration, and curious glances, she receives from others many happy projections of maternal bliss. More important still, the baby within her guarantees in a visible way that she is not empty or without significance. [5]

Other women are more ambivalent about their roles as mother. They feel drained, rather than fulfilled, by having a baby so completely dependent upon them. Especially if a mother chooses to breast feed her child, as she is encouraged by pediatricians and the LaLeche League, she may feel physically and emotionally drained, even entrapped.

Ulanov believes that the ideal relationship between mother and child is one of mutuality, in which child and mother are allowed to experience their own uniqueness, otherness, and yet establish basic trust between themselves:

> A baby needs to know that someone is there who is reliable, friendly, and responsive. A baby also needs to know that he or she is reliably there as a self, worthy of trust and capable of friendliness and responsiveness. Mother and child act and react in mutuality as a working unit, as what D. W. Winnicott calls a "nursing couple." [6]

Earlier I tried to emphasize the mutuality of parental roles in the family unit. In this sense, I consider both parents to be pregnant people, and therefore involved in the adjustments needed to create a family. Basic trust is developed among all, not merely between mother and child. Because of a mother's and child's mutual dependence in breast feeding (when that choice is made), efforts must be made for the father to have intimate time with his child as well. A new mutuality is demanded between the parents as well, to accommodate the demands of a new dependent being in their marriage.

Mastery versus "Making Space"

A woman told of her abashed question to her obstetrician the day after delivery: "Was I just awful during labor?" Seeking reassurance that she "had performed well," she was told, "Well, you weren't the *worst* patient I've ever had!" Her feeling was that she had actually done pretty well at withstanding a difficult and long labor, and wanted to repair any loss of dignity she felt in being overwhelmed and out of control in the process.

In response to the identity crisis mentioned above, there comes a sense of mastery in tension with accommodation. According to Dr. John Grover, Director of the Division of Obstetrics and Gynecology at Lutheran General Hospital, an ideal childbirth experience helps a couple feel as great a sense of mastery as possible. Prepared childbirth classes, provision for birthing rooms, a birthing chair, use of Leboyer techniques for "gentle birth," and sibling visitation all serve to affirm that this is a normal experience, one in which the entire family can take part.

In contrast to this are former views of labor and delivery as being the woman's drama, in which a father could only pace the floor and feel helpless, while the woman passively waited "to be delivered" by her obstetrician. When a woman was overtaken by labor, it is understandable that she would identify with a traditional biblical view of it as a curse, as justifiable punishment by God for her fallenness: "I will greatly multiply your pain in child bearing; in pain you shall bring forth your children. Yet your desire shall be for your husband, and he shall rule over you" (Gen 3:16). If one accepts this view of labor as punishment, then it is seen solely as the woman's burden, rather than as a shared part of a larger fallenness of creation in which both men and women share responsibility for disobedience and alienation from God and each other.

I prefer to understand labor not as punishment, but as a process of mastery and accommodation which enables new life to emerge, much as the beating of the butterfly's wings in the cocoon allows it to strengthen itself enough to fly upon emergence. Mary Maloney Murphy describes it similarly: "Because the birth experience is an intense, short one, she knows in her body the mystery of suffering—joy within a few hours. She experiences pain, but pain in perspective, as only part of a larger, fruitful work."[7]

It is as if the mother's body is preparing for the birth of a baby, making space for it to emerge. Henri Nouwen develops the spiritual concept of hospitality to the events of our lives, "making space" for them rather than fearfully shutting them out and refusing to be influenced by them. Rather than seeing pregnancy, labor, and delivery as interruptions in an otherwise ordered life, we might see them as invitations for hospitality. Space must be made for the development of the child, for the strengthening of the lungs, which happens as the child makes the transition from uterus to world.

Nouwen talks of such "interruptions" as being the very content which gives meaning to our lives, quoting a busy professor as saying:

> You know, my whole life I have been complaining that my work was constantly interrupted, until I discovered that my interruptions *were* my work.[8]

I have been impressed with the way many mothers handle their "interruptions"—the women with incompetent cervices or spontaneous rupture of membranes who are willing to devote months of time to bed rest in hopes that labor will be delayed until their child's lungs mature to the point of surviving birth. For others, the interruption is experienced as hyper-emesis (excessive vomiting, morning sickness) in early pregnancy, at times so severe that it causes a mother to quit work earlier than planned.

Part of mastery is telling the story. In and through such telling and retelling, most women integrate the painful experience of childbirth into the total process. It is almost as if the woman experiences a kind of amnesia in the retelling.

Ulanov sees this storytelling as the creation of an oral tradition that allows a mother to receive the mystery of the child's otherness into her life:

> In such tellings every mother hears variations on the theme of her own experience of the mysterious event of being emerging out of

nothing, of a human person culminating a long, dark interior process foreign to mind and reason. Women gather around a new mother to trade accounts of their version of this mystery. . . . In a process explained biologically and rationally, the altogether wondrous has broken through.[9]

Isolation versus Intimacy

Feeling so helpless when she was hurting, and knowing I could do nothing but put my hand on her or stroke her hair, helped me to know the nakedness of just "being-with" Dawn and knowing it helped with her pain."[10]

Intimacy develops through a mutual journey through a crisis. It is experienced as "a being-with" rather than "a doing-for." Being-with is an acceptance of each individual's responsibility for his or her own life, and a realization of one's lack of control over another person. And yet there comes a sense of closeness between partners-in-labor which allows one to feel fully known, even as God knows us.

> For thou didst form my inward parts,
> Thou didst knit me together in my mother's womb.
> I praise Thee, for Thou art fearful and wonderful.
> Wonderful are Thy works!
> Thou knowest me right well;
> My frame was not hidden from Thee;
> When I was being made in secret,
> Intricately wrought in the depths of the earth.
> (Ps 139:13–15)

The knowledge that God's compassion is with us is sometimes the greatest sense of intimacy and comfort that can be found.

Intimacy is born in the sharing of labor and delivery, between mother and father (or support person), between the couple and their doctor, and also between the parents and child. Being-with described my feelings as I sat with a mother whose bag of waters had broken weeks early — who was awaiting/fearing the development of an infection before her baby's lungs were fully mature. No matter how strong the impulse was to *do* something, to help out, all I could do was to wait it out with her.

A mother who faces a physical crisis might also feel a desperate desire to help her baby's distress, and yet can only "be with" the child as it fights to survive. One mother cried in helpless frustration, "You can't tell me that my child isn't suffering every time I see distress on that fetal heart monitor!"

Justice versus Injustice

> Like a babe stillborn,
> Like a beast with its horns
> I have torn everything
> That touched me.[11]

Cindy was hospitalized for several weeks prior to delivery with diabetes and renal failure. Just two days before her scheduled Caesarean section, she complained about a lack of fetal movement, was examined, and delivered in an emergency procedure. The baby was stillborn, said to have died of a twist in the umbilical cord. Cindy was enraged; the fetus had survived its mother's own serious illness only to die by a fluke — a twist in the cord. She had not wanted any pastoral care prior to delivery; now she was ready to talk with the chaplain. "What kind of a God would allow this to happen?"

In talking with parents in the Compassionate Friends, a parent support group, I find that questions move from "Why me?" to a more resigned "Why not me?" "Why should I be so lucky as to escape?"

Kenneth Moses, a local psychologist who focuses on working with parental grief, talks about this feeling as if one has "lost the magic."[12] Whereas pregnancy and the birth of a baby can awaken a sense of innocence in adults, it can also tap into a deep knowledge of their vulnerability to loss. When a healthy baby is born, parents wonder, "Why are we so lucky?" When a baby is born with problems, parents realize that life is not fair and rage against it. They will never be so innocent again.

Parents in our follow-up grief support group have talked of being six-months pregnant with a subsequent child, and saying, "*If* we have a baby, not *when* we have a baby." They feel hesitant to hope for a healthy child.

Dr. Moses points out that the phase of *rage* in which one says "Why me?" can be a very creative time, one which allows parents to accomplish something in the world to combat the evil they feel encroaching on their lives. They can plant a tree, write letters to doctors, find out autopsy results. The phase of acceptance which realizes "yes, me" allows them to identify with others in similar circumstances and to provide solidarity with them.

Struggle for Immortality versus Surrender to Mystery

> As you do not know how the spirit comes to the bones in the womb of a woman with child, so you do not know the work of God who makes everything. (Eccl 11:5)

Pregnancy, co-creating new life, puts us in touch with awe of creation, no matter what the outcome. Some of my older patients in other parts of the hospital point to their delivery experience as being the one time in their lives they felt closest to God. Childbirth puts us in touch with the mystery of growth, with the amazing rate at which a new baby gains weight and learns new skills. It makes us aware of our profound vulnerability to loss. At the same time that it puts us in touch with a Godlike power to create life, it also reminds us of our finitude.

There is a participation in common human concerns when a mother waits to see whether an infection will develop in her uterus after the bag of waters spontaneously ruptures, or a parent wonders whether one's child will be hit by a car, or whether we will live to see the world destroyed by nuclear warfare.

There is a statement on the wall outside our obstetrics unit in which I would like to take comfort: "Children are God's assurance that life will go on." Maybe so, but under what conditions?

For many parents, there comes a point of surrender. They are aware that, despite the tragedy, one needs to be open to the happy times of the future. One father whose baby died at four and a half months gestation came to our follow-up support group for a year and then, tired of focusing on their sadness, stated: "Yes, I still grieve the loss of our son, but we need to make spaces for the happy times in our lives. We're going to see pain again, too, but I want to be able to enjoy the good times we have."

Pastoral Care Practices

> Give sorrow words; the grief that does not speak whispers the o'er-fraught heart and bids it break.[13]

How do these theological themes and spiritual issues fit into the actual practice of pastoral care with obstetric patients? We chaplains are called into involvement at many points of the childbirth experience, but usually our formalized procedures center around performing baptisms for high-risk infants or at infant deaths, initiating grief responses and paperwork when an infant dies, providing follow-up grief support groups for parents of stillborns and babies who die in neonatal intensive care, offering counseling to those who seek sterilizations or elective abortions.

In general, I view my role as participant and partner with parents, demonstrating a model of God's relationship with them, and their relationship with one another. I qualify this by saying that I do see birth as being a private event, as well as one in which there is a great deal of public interest. My participation is offered with the aim of "making space" for the parent's own needs; my partnership is given with a sense of solidarity with their feelings in the process.

Out of this self-concept, I have developed three working assumptions in my pastoral care of obstetrics patients. Though much of my ministry is to parents of normal deliveries, I must also be available to those parents whose deliveries were abnormal. The following principles are particularly pertinent to that latter group.

A Family-Centered Experience

Whatever is occurring is a family-centered experience, and affects both partners (whether married or not), as well as grandparents and siblings. This first assumption gives rise to the use of birthing rooms and sibling visitation in the case of normal births. Whereas nurses provide a lot of the necessary teaching of breast or bottle feeding, bathing, and self-care, the family will soon assume those tasks, and needs to be valued and affirmed for the support it can offer.

In the case of an infant death, this assumption makes me respectful of the father's as well as mother's style of grieving. Frequently a father becomes fiercely protective, deciding for his wife whether she should see or hold their dead baby. In those cases, I attempt to respond to his grief, rather than immediately assume an advocacy role for the mother. I also am sensitive to the double grief which grandparents experience in a birth crisis: they not only are sad for the illness or death of their grandchild, but also feel helpless to comfort their own child.

Confrontation with Reality

It is important to allow parents to be confronted with the reality of their situation, rather than protected from it. This applies more to crisis ministry than to normal pregnancies. The studies of maternal-infant bonding done by Klaus and Kennell have taught that there is a long-term process of developing dreams prior to the birth of a baby.[14] Parents fantasize about what their baby will look like, will wear, and will be able to do long before the child is delivered. One nurse has referred to the unborn child as the couple's "Gerber baby," perfectly normal, healthy, bouncy, smiling. Whenever anything challenges the parents' fantasy, it constitutes a crisis for the parents. Their "crushed dream" may be as simple as a baby of the opposite gender from their expectations. Or it may be as devastating as a stillbirth or baby with gross anomalies which will allow for survival, but for a very changed child-parent relationship. My frequent question in the grief group for parents of stillborns is, "Who was this child going to be?" Parents usually have an immediate response:

"A sibling. This baby was so important to our four-year-old."

"The completion of our family. It was to be our fourth and last child."

"Our first baby; the first grandchild on both sides. Now my sister-in-law's baby will have that distinction."

"An active athlete like me. You should have felt him kicking!"

Parents have confirmed that it is extremely important that they be offered the opportunity to see their baby, no matter how small. Fantasies about its appearance are usually worse than the reality. I will long remember the parents of a fetus delivered as a late spontaneous abortion, who decided they wanted to see the baby. I have seen dozens of stillborns, and this was about the least recognizably human. It was very small, already in formalin solution. I remember thinking it looked like E.T. I tried to dissuade them from seeing it, but they insisted. Their vision, blinded by their love of this new little dream of theirs, only noticed the perfectly formed fingers, in which they took great comfort.

Importance of Positive Memories
It is important to create positive memories while parents are here, because, for many, these are their only memories of their child outside the womb. The third assumption leads to various procedures for making the birth experience as tangible as possible for parents whose baby will not likely go home with them. I respond to requests for baptism, even of stillborns. One of our students told of an evening on call in which she

was summoned to the emergency room and requested to baptize a woman's dead fetus, presented to her in a brown paper bag. She reported the sense of sacredness both she and the mother felt as she placed the bag on the woman's belly, now so empty, and offered the ritual of baptism.

When baptism is performed, I provide small baptismal gowns sewn by volunteers. A picture is taken of the baby in its gown to reinforce the visual stimuli for a child's parents. A NICU (neonatal intensive care unit) chaplain, writes:

> Meeting recently with parents whose infants had died, we gained a new respect for the significance of the dignity and care associated with the emergency baptismal ritual. For these parents that was the only sacrament that their child would ever receive. The importance of that event cannot be measured or even fully understood by those of us who have never experienced the death of our child.[15]

A complimentary birth certificate, with the baby's footprints on it, is also given to parents, along with a pamphlet, written in consultation with our parents' support group, describing the decisions and feelings to be faced at the death of a child.

Conclusion

My identity and ministry as chaplain on the obstetrics unit has been forged by my experiences listening to women and men as they take part in the creation of new life, and by my own pregnancies and birth-giving process. In my earlier days of training, I disdained the assignment of a woman chaplain to the obstetrics unit, seeing that as stereotyping women in their roles as mother. "Any chaplain should be able to do the job," I thought. My work has had a feminizing influence on me as I realized that it is through my claiming of my own identity as woman and mother that I better understand the struggles of my patients. I have become attuned to women's feelings and images of self, partner, and God. I feel a wholesome sisterhood with those to whom I minister. On a unit with primarily male obstetricians, women value the balance which female nurses and a female chaplain can provide.

However, my awareness of partnership among men and women in creating new life makes me aware of the need for similar connections to be made with the fathers going through these experiences. I encourage the involvement of more male chaplains in this area of ministry so that they might more fully discover their unique contributions in the partnership of pregnancy.

NOTES

1. Mary Murphy, *Creating: Reflections During Pregnancy* (New York: Paulist Press, 1974), p. 34.

2. Lennart Nilsson, *A Child Is Born* (New York: Delacorte Press/Seymour Lawrence, 1977), passim.

3. Nancy Berezin, *Gentle Birth* (New York: Simon and Schuster, 1980), pp. 33–41.

4. A pair of poems by Gordon and Gladis Depree beautifully express this theme: "I am a woman face of God," "I am a man face of God," in Gordon and Gladis Depree, *Faces of God* (New York: Harper & Row, 1974), pp. 62–63.

5. Anne Bedford Ulanov, *Receiving Woman: Studies in the Psychology and Theology of the Feminine* (Philadelphia: The Westminster Press, 1981), p. 99.

6. Ibid., p. 109.

7. Mary Murphy, *Creating: Reflections During Pregnancy* (New York: Paulist Press, 1974), p. 42.

8. Henri J. M. Nouwen, *Reaching Out: The Three Movements of the Spiritual Life* (Garden City: Doubleday and Co., Inc., 1975), pp. 36–37.

9. Ulanov, *Receiving Woman*, pp. 105–106.

10. Tom H. O'Neal, "Theological Reflections on Birth," *Journal of Pastoral Care* 33, no. 4 (December 1979): p. 212.

11. Leonard Cohen, "A Bird on the Wire," cited by Ronna Case, "When Birth Is Also a Funeral," *Journal of Pastoral Care* 32, no. 1 (March 1978): 15.

12. Kenneth Moses, Ph. D., A Lecture to Concerned Parents Organization at Lutheran General Hospital, Park Ridge, Ill. (20 September 1982).

13. Alfred Harbage (ed.), *William Shakespeare The Complete Works*, "Macbeth," Act IV, scene iii (Baltimore: Penguin Books, 1969), p. 1130.

14. Florence Smithe, "Infant Baptism in the Hospital," *The Camillan* 13, no. 2 (February 1981): 9a.

8

The Voices on Pediatrics: Walking with Children and Parents

JIM ARNOLD

Eleven-year-old Tommy was in the hospital for elective surgery. Tommy was a big kid for his age, redheaded, with more than his share of freckles. He was sitting ramrod straight in bed with his eyes locked on the television. "Hi, Tommy. My name's Jim. I'm the chaplain for this unit. What are you watching?" Tommy, his eyes still on the TV, gave a short answer that for all his economy of words, said a lot. The basic message I heard was, "What are you going to do to me?" What Leo Buscaglia says about teachers I believe is true for pastors: "When you start behaving like a 'pastor' in a role, you find yourself saying all kinds of things you wish you hadn't said"[1] — and I did.

I asked him if he knew what a chaplain, pastor, priest, or rabbi was. His answer to each was no. Having backed myself up against a chair, all I could think of was to ask if I could sit down and watch television with him. Tommy agreed and we sat and watched with very little conversation.

During the second commercial break of our session, Tommy favored me by turning his head slightly, focusing his brown eyes on me and saying, "I know what a pastor is. That's the place where they keep the cows." "Okay," I said, "I'd like to be your friend while you're in the hospital." We finally did talk some about surgery (usually at commercial breaks) and about being in the hospital.

His parents arrived and they became the center of attention. I left, going over in my mind what Tommy taught me during our visit. Referring again to Leo Buscaglia and paraphrasing his thoughts about children and teachers, "You know, you are not only a 'pastor,' you are a human being."[2] Children can identify with people, with human beings. They have great difficulty identifying with "pastors."

Children have the same feelings we as adults have, such as fear, lone-liness, guilt, anger, joy, and happiness. A crucial difference is they are still developing life symbols. I wore a white jacket to the hospital one day and not until I had visited three different children, all of whom broke into tears when I entered their rooms, did I realize that the white jacket symbolized a person who was a potential pain-giver. For most children, just coming to the hospital is seen as entering a hostile environment of strange people, frightening and painful experiences, unusual sounds and smells, which require symbols and interpretation.

Usually a mother, transport person, volunteer, or nurse will tell the child, "Now, this is your room and your bed." The minute the child begins to exercise ownership of the room or bed, the realization sets in that the hospital is not "home."

There is a wealth of knowledge related to the effects of illness and hospitalization on children and their families. I need not add a great deal, except to say that effective ministry with hospitalized children, adolescents, and their families comes out of a knowledge and under-standing of their world, particularly of how illness impacts their total life experiences.

Parents are the most important people in a child's world. Therefore, any discussion that speaks of ministry to a child is inadequate and in-complete without placing that ministry within the context of "family." Many times this must include the extended family, grandparents and other relatives, and may need to extend to friends and neighbors. Much of the time ministry goes through the family to the child, especially for the young child and infant.

My young friend at the beginning of this chapter reminded me that ministry is more than religious language and symbols. I agree with Lowell Mays, "Everyone has a spiritual life. Not everyone has a formal religious life."[3] There is a very limiting attitude prevalent in health in-stitutions which identifies patient and family needs for ministry with those who articulate their needs in overtly religious terms. When this happens, usually the chaplain and/or the person's pastor is contacted. To work the implication further, especially for the chaplain, Mays says, "There is a marked distinction between things spiritual and things reli-gious for many people. Some, of course, will see their spiritual life in-cluding the ingredients of religious substance. Others would never in the furthest stretch of their imagination, make a linkage between what is going on in their spirit with a religious commitment."[4]

Hospital ministry is crisis ministry. In a crisis a person's needs are identified in spiritual language — hope, trust, love, and acceptance. For many people the resources to meet these needs may find expression in religious language and symbols. These resources, where present, may be mobilized and affirmed by the chaplain. However, the common resource for all people in crisis is significant: *trustworthy relationships*. This is the dialogue of healing for the human spirit. Perhaps it is ministry with children in crisis which speaks most eloquently to our common needs and forces us beyond roles and systems. It is the theme of this chapter that *the chaplain's mission finds fulfillment through relationships*.

The Prehospital Crisis

For most families, the crisis of a sick child usually begins days before the entrance to the pediatric unit. While many illnesses appear very suddenly, and a child may be perfectly healthy one minute and seriously ill the next, many parents have spent long hours struggling to prevent or stop pain and suffering from overcoming their child. It is during these hours that spiritual needs first begin to be felt in the family.

Basically, most parents want to be "good" parents. The birth of a child brings to mind some old "tapes": "Good parents protect their children from harm"; "Good parents can fix any hurt"; "Good parents are always in control"; "My parents would have done it this way." Before they arrive at the hospital, they are into the spiritual struggle common to us all: *omnipotence versus surrender*. Omnipotence, which troubles us all our lives, becomes a prison whose door we ourselves shut. Freedom is experienced usually as a letting go or as surrender. The need to be not only good parents but perfect ones speaks to the fear of being out of control, of the struggle to accept human limits.

For many parents, their appearance on the pediatric floor represents to some degree both victory and defeat. Victory, in that there is usually some acceptance of their limits as parents and of their ability to protect their child. Behaviorally, parents begin to let go when they make a call to a person they trust and ask for help. This request may produce all manner of suggestions, some of which might work. The physical and spiritual crisis may abate. These same frantic calls to the doctor by those parents whose children are stricken with chronic or life-threatening illnesses can also indicate the exhaustion, frustration, and anger that comes with the months, often years, of living with more questions than answers, or living on the emotional roller coaster of hope and hopelessness.

The Hospitalization Crisis

Arrival at the hospital following their doctor's instructions may be yet a deeper victory over unrealistic parental expectations, acknowledgment that their child needs help of the kind that they as parents cannot provide.

This is a human struggle known to every parent. To acknowledge limitations, to seek help is a victory; however, parents can also feel it as defeat and failure. To compound their troubles, there is the nagging feeling that persists internally and implies personal blame. From my experience, most of the parents who step off the elevators into the hospital world feel guilty and question their own adequacy as caregivers.

Whether their child's hospitalization is due to an accident or a chronic illness, parents must struggle with what it means to be a parent. The meanings of life and their role in the scheme of things are spiritual issues. Parents articulate these meanings in religious (or nonreligious) terms: "God gave me this child" or "I must have done something wrong and God is punishing me" or "I can't understand how God can let this happen to my child." All these questions, and the many others, represent a search for meaning. For many they also represent a collision between their belief systems and the reality of illness, even the possibility of death.

The majority of children who enter the hospital find their stay relatively brief as their illness is successfully treated. For these children, and their families, there may be inconveniences from some sleepless nights and pain from a few shots, but they go home and the experience becomes a "show and tell" next week at school.

Nevertheless, hospitalization is a serious and important experience for every child. It can have both positive and negative results. Children struggling with the anxiety of separation from parents and siblings can gain a sense of mastery in their environment through interaction with a sensitive staff. This interaction often occurs in the child's world of play. A child's fears and misunderstandings of illness and treatment surface in play. The puppets and stuffed animals on our unit have endured a succession of shots. It helped Julie Ann when I showed her in a real syringe just how much blood was to be taken; she has been afraid that they would take all her blood.

I often ask the adolescent patient what it's like to be hospitalized. Frequently, the answer is, "This is weird." This word *weird* seems to describe the awareness that things have suddenly changed—physically, emotionally, and socially. They are in a different environment, removed from the familiar people and surroundings of family, school, and neighborhood. This awareness often induces anxious and negative feelings. For many adolescents, the experience is seen as a time for coping, for getting in, tolerating it, and getting out as quickly as possible. They seem to wade through whatever pain, confusion, and boredom there is and they try to forget the "weird" experience. Other adolescents can be encouraged to use the experience to become more aware of their participation in healthy living. One adolescent girl, because of hospitalization, missed cheerleader tryouts. Her mother was going to talk to the cheerleading coach to try to arrange for a delayed tryout. Through talking with the chaplain, the girl came to realize that she could also make her own needs known and search for ways to solve the problem with the coach herself. The crisis of hospitalization was used positively to continue the development of self-responsibility. For most children and adolescents there is satisfactory adjustment to illness and hospitalization.

Chronic, Life-Threatening Illness

However, when the diagnosis is a chronic and/or life-threatening illness, the world of the family is turned upside down. In these situations the emphasis upon the family as a unit is crucial. Individuals do not resolve stress alone, nor are other members of the family immune from the effects of serious illness. The capacity and strength of some families are awesome as they are asked to rise to their greatest potential at the very time they must face the threat of their greatest loss — the death of their child or the realization that their dream for that child has been shattered by mental deficiencies or physical abnormalities.

Medical science has either eradicated or controlled most of the childhood diseases that in the past claimed children's lives. As a result, the hospital ministry of children and families needs now, and will need with even greater intensity in the future, to focus upon those children with chronic and life-threatening illnesses. If there was ever a question as to the need for ministry to hospitalized children in the past, the fact of medical advances alone makes this ministry mandatory. As many childhood diseases have been conquered, other illnesses, which previously resulted in death, can now be controlled, cured, or remitted, sometimes for long periods.

Advances and possible cures for many children with cancer present both a current and future challenge for care of children and families.

Fourteen years ago, when I began Clinical Pastoral Education, every family whose child was diagnosed with cancer immediately raised for me the question: how can I prepare this family for the death of their child? Today, my first thought is: how can I help them live through the treatments and get on with their lives? Then, the verdict was: your child will die. (Fortunately, some children survived.) Now it is: your child may be cured, and, if not, the chances for long-term survival are increasing. We cannot suspend our concern for continuing growth and development in children until a cure has been proved. Cure must be assumed from the day of diagnosis. We may be proved wrong, but without this attitude, quality of life, whatever its quantity, will be diminished.

When a child in a family is diagnosed with a chronic and/or life-threatening illness, stress multiplies and problems seem insurmountable. The family is threatened and distorted.

The art of crisis intervention is helpful in gaining some perspective for ministry with these children and families. Crisis can be defined as "a change in one's life that produces a modification in perception and relations," or "a change that makes an impact upon the usual life-style of the individual." If we take a longitudinal view, it can be observed that a crisis has both the *potential of danger* (moving toward regression and disintegration) and *of opportunity* (movement toward new learning and integration). *It is also important to recognize that a crisis is both the external situation which provokes it, and the internal response to it.*

The physician, nurse, and medical team members ask how the patient feels. That usually means what is the physical situation in terms of pain, temperature, or other symptoms? These are crucial questions concerning the person's external situation. The answers may necessitate an increase or decrease in medication, a change in treatment.

The chaplain, and other nonmedical caregivers, ask the patient *what* they are feeling in order to focus upon their internal response to the external precipitant. Such responses have important bearing upon one's values, beliefs, and relationships.

This interplay between diagnosis and medical treatment, and the emotional and spiritual response to both, determines how a child and family moves through a crisis.

"Serious illness," as Kenneth Vaux points out, "especially in children, poses the basic question of theodicy: Is there a God? If so, does He care? If He cares, why does He allow this apparent evil? Is it in some way our fault or within our power to prevent."[5] He goes on to state that one of the answers is found in the Twenty-third psalm. "I fear no evil; for Thou art with me." God is with us even when many times we do not feel His presence. God's presence is felt most vividly through persons who walk alongside. *Ministry then becomes walking with children and their parents through the journey of testing, diagnosis, treatment, perhaps relapse, even death.*

Admission

First, ministry means identifying soon after admission those families whose responses to diagnosis and treatment suggest possible trouble. It is during this initial period that those symptoms or issues need to be identified and shared with the staff. Family members need the opportunity to ventilate their fears and anxieties. Parents need affirmation as caregivers of their child. They need assurance of their continued importance in decision making and in the daily care of their child.

Diagnosis Is Confirmed

The time waiting for test results is when time stands still. Tests and diagnosis are a crucial second stage. Suspicions and fears may already be present; however, until a firm diagnosis is made, families are held in suspension. This is usually the time when fantasies, usually bad, plague parents.

Children undergo painful spinal taps, blood drawing, upper and lower gastrointestinal tests, sometimes exploratory surgery and more. Waiting for results brings feelings of helplessness and impotence flooding to the surface. During this phase, families need reassurance, presence, prayers of their faith community, and the chance for reflection. Staff can encourage this difficult but necessary process.

When the diagnosis confirms the worst fears, we have found it helpful for the chaplain to be present with the physician and family for the explanation and treatment outline. One father expressed the need for a chaplain by explaining that "something is given birth during that conference." Shock, fear, anger, disbelief—all these feelings, he said, "need someone to attend to the afterbirth." This father was identifying the nonmedical concerns common to all families at the time of diagnosis. These families look to their physicians to lead and manage the medical aspects of their child's treatment. They should also be able to look to the chaplain, to give guidance in developing a support system through the treatment process.

Many times families do not hear any words after being told that their son or daughter has a neuroblastoma, leukemia, or one of the other childhood cancers. *This is a time when both parents should be present.* Usually this conference with the parents should be held apart from the child, particularly with preteenaged children. This gives the physician, chaplain, and parents an opportunity to plan together how to tell the child.

I cannot overemphasize the importance of this initial physician-family conference. It has been suggested that both individual and family reactions to threats are fashioned in the early weeks, usually within the first four weeks, following the confirmation of the diagnosis.[6] Also, it is during those initial days that relationships between the child/family and the professionals begin to form. The chaplain's task becomes one of being alert to these dynamics and becoming a facilitator of their expression. Two factors enhance the fulfillment of this role: first, the chaplain is seen by staff and family as nonmedical; and second, most people recognize that relationships are central to the chaplain's mission.

It has been my experience that for many chronic illnesses, early intervention by a nonmedical professional is important in facilitating the difficult coping process. The chaplain often has the opportunity to become the nonmedical professional who remains constant during the weeks, months, or years of repeated hospitalizations.

The physician-chaplain relationship is a key to making this happen in the hospital. Through mutual respect and collegiality, these professionals working together convey a powerful message to newly diagnosed families. The combination of physician and chaplain promises medical treatment (cure or control) for the disease and sensitive care for their responses to the disease.

Patients (and parents) seem to remember little of what doctors tell them, particularly when initial anxiety or denial reactions prevail. One of the early stresses for these families is to go home the first night after diagnosis and to telephone grandparents and friends to repeat what the doctor said. The emotional trauma of their own feelings is now compounded by the real or imagined reactions of others. Blockage of many details explained by the physician is understandable. We at Lutheran General Hospital have instituted audiotaping of the initial conference, and also the session where the protocol for the child's treatment is detailed. The family is given the audiotape and has the opportunity to share it with extended family or friends. They also can go back over the conversation themselves and begin the arduous process of working through their feelings and implementing the agreed-upon plans.

Treatment Begins

The initial treatment phase becomes the next traumatic experience for the child/family. For those children newly diagnosed with diabetes, this time requires not only dealing with the emotional reactions — sorting through myths and facts about future life-styles — but also a time of intense education. Learning about the disease and how the body reacts, how to use food exchanges and to give insulin shots, becomes crucial to successful living. Children starting treatment for cancer begin dealing with the side effects of chemotherapy, radiation therapy, or both. Particularly for the older child and the adolescent, the loss of hair can become the most devastating side effect. For many of these kids, this affects them more than the life-threatening possibility. Adolescents are at a time in life when appearance to their peers is very important. Any assault on their body threatens an already fragile self-image.

Parents of adolescent patients have unique needs. Whereas parents of younger children must struggle with the full responsibility for making decisions on behalf of their dependent children, parents of the teenager must deal with growing independence. In one of our parent support groups, parents often discuss the agony of making life-and-death decisions when they have younger children versus parents of adolescents who must surrender control and cope with their teenager's decision to terminate chemotherapy.

From the beginning, parents of these children fear the threat of death. Expressions of these fears vary as individuals vary. Some parents express their fears and anxieties openly, while others suffer in silence and resist any offer of support. Fathers and mother also react as individuals. One parent may be open while the other is very closed. Here again, the important parent-physician conference assists parents to hear the same information at the same time. When the mother is alone for the conference, she has the responsibility of relaying the information to her husband. Second-hand information is inadequate at best; as well, the mother has to deal with the father's emotional responses and field his questions. When both parents are present, the health professionals can become positive role models for them in the art of communication. Such an occasion also gives opportunity to discuss ways and means parents can fulfill their caring role, even during hospitalization.

During this initial week or two it becomes helpful to identify some important relationships, specifically parents and children who are on the same journey. While each family and each individual within the family is unique, a common experience enables strangers to say to one another:

I know how you feel. This was dramatically brought into focus in the room of a seventeen-year-old male with leukemia. We had arranged for a seven-year old with a similar disease to visit him. They both had lost their hair from treatments and the younger boy was very troubled about this. It was beautiful to observe these two young people as they hesitantly began to talk. The subject of hair loss and wigs came up and the older boy showed his wig to the younger one. They talked about how strange the wigs felt and even commented on how they smelled. Some weeks later at a memorial service for the seventeen-year-old, the mother of the young boy said that the earlier visit had given her son something no one else could — *the awareness that he was not alone.*

Leaving the Hospital

After families leave the hospital, many return for out-patient treatments. Once again the assurance of availability and support, a continued "walking with," becomes important. Often, relationships with another family have been established. Between clinic visits and hospitalizations, parents report a multitude of daily living concerns that can best be met by face-to-face or telephone fellowship with other families. The chaplain's role in bringing these families together extends that ministry beyond personal presence.

When families have a faith group, the chaplain can become a bridge between the hospital world and that community. The chaplain may also have the opportunity to be involved with these families in support groups. In mutual support or self-help groups, the focus is usually on concerns and problems of daily living. Often, the group can provide a place where parents and/or children will feel comfortable enough to talk about their problems. Together these families begin to discover and develop strengths and resources.

Barbara Sourkes lists four areas of intervention helpful to families with a child undergoing treatment for cancer.[7] I believe they are equally applicable for all chronic life-threatening illnesses in children. They are:

1. *Facilitation of Communications*
   "Helping individuals convert the 'implicit' to the 'explicit,' allowing for clearer communication of feelings and needs."

2. *Ongoing Availability*
   "Availability is not calculable; it cannot be assessed through number of hours spent . . . rather, availability is a subjective

construct whose meaning derives from a recognized mutuality
. . . an abiding trust."

3. *Giving Permission*

"To express ambivalent feelings, a respect for the individual 'pacing' or allowing people into family space when they are ready."

4. *Modeling of Skills for the Parent*

"Care-giving and coping skills or helping parents to be the kind of parents to their child they want and need to be." The dialogue of healing is a covenant or a commitment one to the other. With support, most families do survive the crisis, forever changed but together.

Throughout the treatment process some children may approach death and then rally for extended periods of time. During such times the chaplain once again has the responsibility of walking with the family. Each of these crises reproduces all the original feelings of helplessness, anger, fear, and sadness. These agonizing feelings are added to the stress and strain of treatments and tests. Not only is the family thrust once again toward despair when a relapse occurs; they may be in jeopardy when the child is in remission. When a child approaches death, the family begins anticipatory mourning, that is, they begin emotionally experimenting with what their future will be like without the child. When, as sometimes happens, the child recovers, or at least does so for a period of time, it is as if the child returned from the dead. William Easson refers to this as the "Lazarus syndrome."

The child who recovers from an illness that is usually fatal may return to his family as if he were a new family member. His parents, his brothers and sisters and close relatives have the difficult emotional task of adapting to this new and unexpected person. The dying child can never recover and be seen again as the child he was before. When Lazarus returns from the grave, he comes back not as the beloved brother, but as the stranger who has to become known and hopefully to become loved.[8]

It is important, particularly for staff, to stay in touch with the tremendous emotional conflict produced by both good and bad news.

When Death Comes

In their wonderful book *Children Die, Too,* Joy and Marv Johnson tell about a statue in the Mormon cemetery in Omaha, Nebraska. "Two pioneer parents stand over the open grave of their child, their heads close together—winter wind billowing their capes as the father's hand holds his shovel."[9] When we allow ourselves to think about death, there is the assumption of a rhythm in life. The expectation is that children bury their parents. As Barbara Sourkes puts it:

> The child who is dying throws a certain assumed sequence out of order. We expect a time in life when a reversal of roles will occur, when children will care for dying parents. When parents find themselves watching a child die instead, there is a constant sense of tragic absurdity. Not only is time shortened, but its order is upset. A dying child represents a premature separation to the family. Even before the child has become a differentiated individual through the natural developmental process of separation, the child is wrenched away by death. We have little rehearsal for separation by death, and even less when a psychological separation has not been effected.[10]

Ministry to the dying child and family once again emphasizes time. How much time do we have? Of course, we never know.

Working in a hospital brings staff face to face with sudden death as when a child is hit by a car or comes through the emergency room having fallen into the backyard swimming pool or nearby pond. An infant may be admitted and die within a few hours. The final diagnosis may be a "sudden infant death syndrome." These and other fatal times bring together a grief-stricken family and a pediatric staff, and we are all strangers to each other. The chaplain moving into this life-and-death drama encounters the whole range of human emotions from, "Stay away from me, I don't need a chaplain, my child's not going to die," to parents who agonizingly request that their child be baptized and want an immediate call placed to their clergy.

The goal of ministry remains focused on relationships. The chaplain must move quickly, but gently into the drama of medical technology, highly skilled physicians, nurses, and technicians, and into an adjoining room that houses weeping and grief-stricken parents awaiting the final verdict. There may only be a wall separating them; however, the chaplain once again must move between two worlds.

The capacity and skill to move confidently from one world to another gives value and meaning to the presence of the chaplain. At few other times does the chaplain's symbolism become so important. This is as valuable to the staff as it is to the family. All involved become conscious of the need for a power greater than themselves. Probably the question most asked of the staff by the chaplain is: is there any word I can give the family? Any word from the world where the child is struggling for life helps to sustain the parents for a few more minutes. One of the greatest needs of parents at this time is to be with or near their child. Words from the chaplain who has been with their child may be as close as they can get, at least for now.

Though parents often cannot remain in the treatment area, they should be given as much time as possible to be with and to hold their child. I often encourage parents as they sit holding their baby or young child to talk about those dreams they have had since before the birth of the child. All parents begin to dream dreams for their expected child. When the actual or threatened loss intrudes into their lives, *it is the anticipated need to bury dreams that becomes unbearable.* Many of these dreams have never been verbalized and parents can experience some relief when encouraged to share these, even when their child is in a coma.

After the child has died, parents still need to share shattered hopes and dreams. It is a necessary part of mourning. Such sharing helps give one the courage and permission to say goodbye.

Anticipatory grieving begins for parents when a potenially fatal diagnosis is made. For many this is at a very deep level, sometimes without verbalization. Usually, if the child dies, a parent may realize that the burying of dreams had been going on inside for a long time.

Ministry to families who experience the death of a child must continue after the death. If possible, it is important to link the family to their own clergy throughout the illness. A chaplain is much like a pediatric subspecialist: the intersecting with a family is brief, during the heat of the crisis. It is the attending physician and parish clergy who provide the ongoing care. However, on occasion, the chaplain's ministry to a specific family may continue both directly and indirectly.

Whatever the period of time involved, the family and health care staff have been on a journey together. Just as families anticipate the death of their child, the staff experiences that death. The chaplain's freedom to move into the worlds of both the staff and family, intervening and supporting, is vital. Following the death of a child, the staff may choose to attend the funeral services with the family. Or, a special time for the staff to gather and share their grief with one another may be encouraged by the chaplain.

Following the death of their child, the message that most families give to the staff who cared for their child is that their child was very special to them. In some way, they hope that their child was special to the staff. Every staff person, but especially those close to the family, needs to communicate to them that the child was special and will not be forgotten.

The ministry to these families may also include making a referral to a parents' group, such as the Compassionate Friends, which has chapters in most communities. Many chaplains serve as facilitators for grief groups in their hospitals and many then have the opportunity for an extended ministry. It may also be helpful to be available to the parents and siblings for several postdeath conferences, especially those families who do not have the support of an extended family and/or clergy. Walking with these children and their families, living and dying, is a ministry through relationships that is both critical and rewarding for the chaplain.

The dialogue for healing (as the word *dialogue* implies) is a giving and receiving. The communication process is not complete until the receiver has been not only heard but also understood. Dialogue of healing also means that we as health care professionals are sometimes the healers and often, the healed. The gift that children and families give is the privilege to enter their world of pain and illness and to walk alongside. And in that journey, our own lives are enriched and blessed.

NOTES

1. Leo Buscaglia, *Living, Loving and Learning* (New York: Rinehart and Winston, 1982), p. 8.

2. Ibid.

3. Lowell H. Mays, "Spirituality: A Concern for Health and Cancer Support," *Proceedings of the American Cancer Society*, Third National Conference on Human Values and Cancer, Washington, D.C., 1981, p. 117.

4. Ibid.

5. Kenneth Vaux, "Laurie's Story," *Living with Childhood Cancer*, ed. J. Spinetta et al. (St. Louis, Mo.: C. V. Mosby Co., 1981), p. 74.

6. David M. Kaplan, "Family Mediation of Stress Posed by Severe Illness" (Unpublished Paper).

7. Barbara Sourkes, "Facilitating Family Coping with Childhood Cancer," *Journal of Pediatric Psychology* 2, no. 2 (February 1977): 65-67.

8. William M. Easson, *The Dying Child* (Springfield: C.C. Thomas, 1970), p. 80.

9. J. Johnson and S. M. Johnson, *Children Die, Too* (Council Bluffs, Iowa: Centering Corporation, 1978), p. 2.

10. Sourkes, "Facilitating Family Coping," pp. 65-67.

9

The Voices on a Surgery Unit:
The Loss of Control

MARION KANALY

A student nurse makes a referral to the surgical chaplain. "Could you talk to Mrs. Brown? She's very depressed. She cries all the time." The chaplain inquires further, and it becomes apparent that the referring nurse is uncomfortable with the patient's tears. She expects the chaplain to get the patient to feel less depressed (that is, to stop crying), or even better, to cheer her up completely.

While the patient in this situation is certainly someone who may be helped by the chaplain's ministry, possibly the more immediate pastoral task is to spend a few moments with the nurse: a time to draw her out, to explore her reaction to patients who cry or otherwise appear "down," a time to do some informal teaching about depression as a valid dynamic in the context of illness and surgery.

Joe is a new patient on the surgical floor and scheduled for a TUR (Trans-urethral resection). During a presurgical pastoral call, Joe demonstrates considerable anxiety. His body language is expressive. His hands are in constant motion, he turns and twists on the bed. Yet Joe smiles and jokes in a way that seems incongruent with his admission of feeling "scared." On this initial visit, Joe cannot seem to identify the cause for such feelings. It is only later that Joe shares with the chaplain his fear of aging. That is what scares him. Joe is fifty-four. Except for the usual childhood illnesses, he has always enjoyed excellent health. All of a sudden his body is starting to show the wear and tear of those fifty-four years. Is this the beginning of a downhill slide, he wonders?

Rosalie is thirty years old and four and a half months pregnant with her first child. But something seems to have gone wrong. Certain symptoms point toward a miscarriage, yet the first ultrasound reveals a fetal heartbeat. After thirty-six hours of complete bed rest, the symptoms persist. A second ultrasound, however, shows no sign of fetal life, and Rosalie's obstetrician thinks it is time to consider a pregnancy termination.

Rosalie is deeply distressed by that recommendation for two reasons: she and her husband want this baby very much, and they are Roman Catholics. She is very fearful and tearful. As the hours pass, she can only focus on one question: how can God ever forgive her if she agrees to abort the pregnancy?

Walter, ninety years old, was admitted to the surgical floor from the emergency room with a probable leg fracture. Six months previously he had made a successful recovery from surgery for a fractured pelvis. But the trauma of a broken hip and the lengthy rehabilitation process wrought significant behavioral changes in Walter. From being independent, active, and alert — in spite of his years — he became more and more forgetful and confused, and was moved into a convalescent home. Now he was back in the hospital. During the first forty-eight hours, while X rays and tests were being done, Walter became increasingly disturbed. He was noisy, repetitious, and disoriented.

His daughter and son-in-law spent many hours at his bedside trying to calm him. The daughter was distressed and "embarrassed" (her word). Attentive, loving, and patient with her father, she felt badly because he was so difficult for the nurses. She kept apologizing for his behavior. She stayed late into the night with him and returned early the next morning. Her presence was welcomed by the staff for its quieting effect on the patient and because she was a real help in his care. However, staff was concerned that she would get overtired and overstressed.

John, single, sixty years old, is scheduled for a femoral bypass (a surgical procedure to insert a graft around an obstruction of the femoral artery). Before the surgery can be done, a number of tests must be performed, so John is here for several days before the operation. He has no family except for some cousins who live in a distant state. He lives in a rented room in a private home whose owners are concerned about him. He has also been befriended by the minister of a local church. Apart from these few individuals, John has no significant support system. He is very apprehensive about the surgery but unable to verbalize his feelings. At his doctor's request, the chaplain spends considerable time with John each day, and though John never says a lot, he seems to appreciate her visits.

Pauline went into surgery at 1:00. It is now 5:30 and her husband, sister, and brother-in-law are still in the family surgical lounge. They had been told the operation would take only one and a half to two hours, but they have had no word of Pauline's status for four and a half hours. Earlier in the afternoon the chaplain had visited with the family. They were fairly relaxed. Now on this return visit they are extremely anxious and distraught. Why the long delay? Does it mean something has gone wrong? The surgeon had seemed so positive it would be an uncomplicated procedure. Can the chaplain find out what's going on?

These are but a few of the voices encountered by a chaplain on the general surgical floor of a large teaching hospital. The voices illustrate something of the broad range of pastoral ministry: *to staff, to patients, to families.* They also illustrate something of the range of needs and dynamics that can surface in the world of the surgical patient.

With the student nurse, ministry is a combination of teaching and challenge. It is directed at helping her to enlarge her capacity for understanding a patient with whom she shares little except common humanity. Her patient, Mrs. Brown, is eighty-five years old. Except for times of childbirth she has never been hospitalized in her long life. This is an alien world for her. Her nurse is twenty years old, two-thirds of the way through nursing school. The hospital is a familiar, comfortable world for her. It is not too surprising that there is a gap of understanding as big as there is in years of living between nurse and patient.

Mrs. Brown has felt lonely and lost many times during the past ten days while undergoing all kinds of tests and work-ups. At last, her doctor tells her that exploratory surgery is necessary. Mrs. Brown is frightened: of the unknown, of the decision *she* must make, of growing old, and of an illness that may mean she can no longer care for herself as she has done until now. Ministry to Mrs. Brown must be supportive. Its goal is to comfort her by being present to her and by encouraging her to identify some of her own coping strengths gained from a rich treasure of life experiences.

For Joe there is also fear. A TUR can reveal cancer of the prostate. What if it turns out that he does have that dreaded disease? If so, will he have to change or adjust his life-style? Will he have to forego achieving some of the personal and vocational goals he still envisions?

At first, during earlier pastoral visits, Joe claimed that his apprehension was related to growing older. When he began to absorb the implications that surgery might expose a malignancy, he discovered how fragile health and well-being are, and how suddenly a person can go from feeling normal and healthy to being at risk of serious illness. Ministry to Joe involved supporting his struggle to adjust to some new realities. It meant encouraging him to verbalize the questions that were churning around in his mind. In meant to be with him, challenging him when appropriate to search out his own responses, identify his own personal values and strengths, look at what gives him a sense of worth and purpose in his life.

In contrast, ministry with Rosalie focused much more explicitly on some basic religious-theological issues, primarily those of guilt, forgiveness, and God's grace.

Rosalie's sense of guilt had little, if anything, to do with feeling she was to blame somehow for the failure of her pregnancy. Hers was an anticipated guilt: that by consenting to a necessary therapeutic pregnancy termination she would be contravening divine law, as she perceived the Roman Catholic position on abortion. In her emotional and spiritual distress Rosalie was unable to distinguish the finer points of her church's teaching. Nor could she hear the wise counsel of her physician, himself a member of that church. The chaplain's role here was twofold: to assure Rosalie that God's forgiveness was hers as a gift of grace and to call in (with her permission) a Roman Catholic priest who was able to explain that no sin was involved in her giving consent to a surgical termination of the pregnancy.

Many times it is the family of a patient who is more in need of ministry. Such was the case with Walter. Walter himself was too disoriented to enter into a shared relationship. The chaplain could do little except sit with him and hold his hand, trying to convey both verbally and nonverbally some comfort that might alleviate his distress. It was his daughter who needed assurance and acceptance. She expressed embarrassment at the trouble she thought her father was causing the staff and other patients. It was important to enable her to talk out her feelings and concerns, but also to affirm that her father's behavior was not uncommon, given his age and the trauma he was experiencing. The staff understood the situation, and they appreciated her willingness to help with his care.

Ministry to John was mostly a matter of presence and the expression of personal concern for a lonely person who had a very limited support system. When John went for an angiogram (an X ray procedure which injects contrast materials into the blood vessels to determine disease and/or an obstruction of blood flow), the chaplain accompanied him. On the day of surgery the local minister was invited to join the chaplain in accompanying John to the operating room and in meeting him later in the recovery room. Through the initiative of that minister some appropriate visitors from the congregation were mobilized to visit John during his postsurgical hospital stay.

One of the important settings for crisis ministry is the family surgical lounge where relatives wait while their loved one is in surgery. This is a stressful time for families. Minutes seem like hours and hours like days, especially when the surgery exceeds the estimated time frame. That is what happened with Pauline.

Fortunately, the chaplain has access to the surgical control desk and can request that staff call the surgical suite to discern the status of the patient, or even speak on the phone to a member of the surgical team. In this way it was possible to learn that Pauline's surgery had been late in starting, which partially accounted for the long delay, and that the surgeon had wanted to have some extra tests done before finishing the operation. The surgeon advised the chaplain to tell the family that Pauline was doing very well and that her husband would be able to go into the recovery room to see her shortly.

Emotional Needs

Coming to the hospital as a patient has different meanings for each person, but for just about everyone there is some feeling of apprehension. Even for those who have had a previous hospitalization, there is an element of uncertainty. The prospect of surgery adds to the stress. The overarching emotional dynamic is fear. When invited to explore such feelings, many surgical patients describe it as a fear of nonbeing, a fear of death. They are afraid they won't make it. They focus on fear of the anesthesia, which seems to be a symbol of nonbeing, of going into the uttermost depths of the unknown from which they may never again emerge. Most of us who are healthy believe we will stay that way. There are relatively few of us who believe we will contract a serious disease or require major surgery. Intellectually we know that permanent good health is not a guarantee. Emotionally we feel that illness and surgery happen only to other people, not to us.

Being (or feeling) out of control is a corollary dynamic of the basic fear and anxiety that surgical patients experience. It is an unfortunate, although necessary, fact of hospitalization that all patients lose some degree of control over their lives. They must give up their own clothes and put on hospital attire. They eat when meal trays come, whether or not they feel hungry. They have to share their living space with others. Real privacy is rare. Doctors, nurses, technicians, therapists, and yes, chaplains too, along with visitors and the volunteer with the book cart, come and go from the room at *their* convenience, not the patient's. All of this is with good purpose, but patients have to tolerate the constant intrusions into their space.

In addition to the loss of control, *the person going to surgery knows that life itself is about to be managed and ordered totally by others for a period of time. Here is the ultimate and absolute loss of control over oneself.* Heartbeat and breath will be maintained through the direction of other people, not the *I* who hitherto has been in charge.

For some patients the issue of control causes no significant problems. There are those patients, however, for whom the hospital setting and system generate excessive dependency. Some react with irritability, resistance, or hostility. Others seek to keep some shred of control by maintaining an attitude of detachment, withholding permission for staff to engage them at a personal level.

Unfortunately, and all too often, such behavior can lead to stereotyping or labeling the patient by the staff. To be dependent is to be "manipulative." To be irritable is to be "resistant." To be quiet is assessed as "withdrawal" or "depression." Patients who ask questions about their medications or prescribed procedures are perceived as "overanxious" or "hostile." Such assessments carry with them suggestions of emotional pathology in the patient.

By no means is this labeling done with negative or malicious intent. Most health care givers are genuinely kind and concerned people. They want their patients to get well, to feel good, to be healed. This is more than a "want," it is often *a deep need* of the care provider. And it is an appropriate need, but its fulfillment is found too often in "cure" rather than in truly empathetic care. In so doing, staff will then look for demonstrable proof that the patient is "really getting better," as evidenced by a cheerful spirit, compliance, and a willingness to engage in social conversation or self-disclosure.

At a recent staffing on one of our surgical units the status of two patients was reviewed. The two men shared the same room; both had undergone surgery. I was asked if I knew why Anthony was so depressed. When I inquired of the reporting nurse why she thought this man was depressed, she replied that it was because he did not talk much, slept a lot, and was quiet. In actuality, Anthony was simply a quiet person. He was reticent about sharing personal feelings, and his wife confirmed in a conversation that he had always been this way. Even so, the nurse was still convinced that the patient was depressed. She compared him with his roommate who was very gregarious, open, and talkative. To be like that was, in the nurse's mind, to be truly healthy and together. Because

Anthony was a different personality, she felt there must be some emotional imbalance.

Through such stereotyping a patient may be cut off from needed support, thereby increasing a sense of "existential loneliness," which Clark E. Moustakas defines as a state of being "fully aware of oneself as an isolated and solitary individual."[1] The surgical patient confronts existential loneliness in a real way. *It is the patient who goes alone into the experience.* There are many other people around, but for all their care and help and encouragement, it is the patient who alone submits to the surgeon's scalpel. That is a very lonely place to be. Reflecting postoperatively on the experience, one woman told me: "When they came to wheel me into the operating room and I said goodbye to my husband and daughter, I couldn't stop thinking that this must be what dying is like. You're so alone. No one can do it for you. No one can go through it with you, not really."

Along with such experiences as loss of control and some loss of personal identity, the surgical patient often has to cope with other kinds of losses, some temporary, some permanent. Most immediately, there is a loss of mobility. It is difficult for a person who has been reasonably, or even moderately, active to accept that getting out of bed, taking a shower, caring for fundamental physical needs, walking into the hall, should be done with assistance from a nurse or health aide. This diminished freedom to move around independently is often further complicated by medical apparatus, such as an IV, a catheter, a nasogastric tube, an oxygen mask, or the like.

For the majority of surgical patients these limitations will only be temporary. For others, however, some type of loss may be permanent. When this occurs, the person must begin to cope with the threatening dynamics of irreversible change.

This is so for the woman whose breast cancer requires a mastectomy. She faces a threatening change in her self-image.

She may face the threat of change in her relationships: with her husband, if married; with male friends and female friends; with members of her family and colleagues at work. How will all these relationships go now? Will other people find it awkward to be at ease in her presence? What about her relationship with herself? What about threatening changes in her self-perception? What changes in her day-to-day life, her life-style, her beliefs and ideas about her personhood and where her sense of personhood is grounded, in her hopes, dreams, and goals for the future?

Such questions are often harsh and painful. A permanent loss, whether or not it is connected to a life-threatening disease, is likely to generate complex emotional experiences. Of course, each person's reactions will be unique. The nature of the response will depend in part on that individual's prior experiences of loss or unwanted change, and how those experiences were handled. And much—perhaps everything—will depend upon the individual's own system of beliefs. Paul Tillich referred to these as "ultimate concern." By that he meant the set of core beliefs or values upon which we center our lives and which are the basis for our understanding of the essential meaning of life.

It is this ultimate concern, as apprehended subjectively, which helps or hinders a person in responding to all the other concerns that accompany such life's experiences.

Pastoral Response to the Voices: Koinonia as Hospitality and Healing

> . . . creating space is far from easy in our occupied and preoccupied society. And still, if we expect any salvation, redemption, healing and new life, the first thing we need is an open receptive place where something can happen to us. . . . We cannot . . . change other people by our convictions, stories, advice and proposals, but we can offer a space where people are encouraged to disarm themselves, to lay aside their occupations and preoccupations and to listen with attention and care to the voices speaking in their own center.[2]

The concept of hospitality, shaping what Nouwen calls "an open, receptive place where something can happen," is central to my ministry on a surgical floor. Hospitality, in this sense, begins with openness to the patient, the family member, the staff person, to whomever my ministry is directed. It begins with the offer of a relationship that the other is free to accept or not accept. To use a theological image, it is the offer of a covenant between myself and the other, symbolically modeling the divine-human encounter wherein God invites each human being to enter into a personal relationship, which both respects and affirms the freedom of each party.

In extending a similar kind of invitation to the hurting person, I want to communicate not only my personal concern, but God's concern for that individual, and at the same time to leave space for the other to be free in choosing how to respond. Creating, or trying to create, that open space is especially important in the hospital setting, which by its very nature tends to place many restrictions on individual freedom.

Objectively, the purpose of such restrictions is appropriate and reasonable. But there is a subjective side as well which needs to be considered. The majority of hospital patients today have a broader awareness of health matters and a more acute sensitivity to themselves as persons — not cases — than may have been true a generation ago. On the whole, they expect to be treated both as reasonably intelligent and as feeling human beings. When they experience respect for those qualities in themselves, they are fortified to engage more effectively in their own healing process.

However, if comments by patients are fairly accurate expressions of how they perceive the realities of the hospital world, it appears that many do not experience respect for themselves as persons. In many ways, they see themselves being "objectified." Those responsible for their care often fail to communicate well, or so patients say. Patients feel the lack of clear information or explanation of procedures as a lack of interest in them as unique persons.

Granted, professional health care workers are very busy people who cannot be expected to spend long periods of time with each individual patient. Granted also, not all of them are impersonal in their attitudes. Yet there is much that happens in the day-to-day experience of the hospital that in effect causes the patient to feel more like *an object* to which things are done than a unique human being who is accorded the space to participate in what is being done.

It is the rich opportunity of the chaplain to help counterbalance these "objectified" aspects of illness, surgery, and the hospital experience, by reshaping the environment to allow the patient to feel some open space whereby she or he can be known in a personal way. As a chaplain I come to the patients on my unit making few demands. I come to offer a caring presence, an assurance of acceptance, a reminder of the divine presence and acceptance of the one who is for both the patient and myself Creator, Redeemer, Sustainer, the Ultimate Source of all that we are in our shared humanity. I come to learn from, as well as to do for: to learn from the other what it is like to be in that hospital bed, to confront the threats and limits of suffering, to learn as much about that person as the other wishes to disclose.

That is the first stage of the relationship between us. Sometimes it goes no further because the patient feels no need to go further. *Not everyone needs a chaplain.* Yet just about all of us, simply because we're human, need, or at least value, some expression of interest in ourselves. To some degree we all have a deep yearning for acceptance. To experience acceptance helps us to cope with those common human feelings of alienation and brokenness that are an integral part of being human.

The surgical patient who has encountered fear of the unknown (including fear of death); fear of irreversible changes and permanent limitations; a sometimes bewildering and overwhelming number of losses; and considerable physical and psychic pain, will crave acceptance without strings attached. Most likely such patients will not respond to a smooth, condescending approach which fails to honor their unique personhood, but will respond to a relationship that recognizes the bond of common and shared humanness.

The concept of *koinonia* (a Greek word meaning "community" or "assembly") comes to mind as a way of describing what I seek to cultivate through pastoral ministry in the hospital. There is, of course, the kerygma to be proclaimed, the good news of God's reconciling love and boundless grace. More often than not, in fact most of the time, this kerygmatic function is done by implication in the hospital context. Koinonia is more directly expressed by communicating to the patient a sense of belonging, of being gathered in, of being part of a community, whether that be the faith community as usually understood, or the broader community of humankind.

The caring, empathic, healing community that enfolds the patient is koinonia. Part of the pastoral response is to be one who helps shape this community, whether in one-to-one encounters with patients and staff, embracing the patient and family, serving as an informal advocate for the patient within the hospital, or providing a link to the patient's spiritual resources and support system after hospitalization. Whatever the particular context of each situation, my aim is to walk beside the other in a shared relationship that imitates in microcosm the New Testament image of the "beloved community," where redemption and healing and reconciliation might be dynamically available to those who enter it. In this regard, Henri Nouwen's thoughts on hospitality merit attention:

> Hospitality, therefore, means primarily the creation of a free space where the stranger can enter and become a friend instead of an enemy. Hospitality is not to change people, but to offer them space where change can take place. It is not to bring men and women over to our side, but to offer freedom not disturbed by dividing lines. It is not to lead our neighbor into a corner where there are no alterna-

tives left, but to open a wide spectrum of options for choice and commitment. . . . It is not a method of making our God and our way into the criteria of happiness, but the opening of an opportunity to others to find their God and their way. The paradox of hospitality is that it wants to create emptiness, not a fearful emptiness, but a friendly emptiness where strangers can enter and discover themselves as created free; free to sing their own songs, speak their own languages, dance their own dances.[3]

Within that "friendly emptiness," there can be space for many pastoral responses. In a way, recovery from surgery is like "a resurrection experience." The gift of life is renewed, a gift to celebrate and rejoice in—patient and chaplain—together.

Whether recovery is complete or only partial and temporary, there is an opportunity to explore some important questions with patients. What have they learned about themselves from this experience, about their own ways of coping, their own strengths? What, if anything, has been sacred about it? Has it caused them to think any differently about their life values and priorities? Beyond the physical pain and emotional stress, beyond any loss suffered, is there a sense of hope and promise, and in what way?

In our hospital the average length of stay for surgical patients is about six to eight days. For many the time is shorter; for a few it may be much longer. So it may not always be possible to address fully the kinds of questions and issues mentioned above. Still, issues can be lifted up by name, if nothing else, and perhaps some seeds of reflection planted.

NOTES

1. Clark E. Moustakas, *Loneliness* (Englewood Cliffs, N. J.: Prentice-Hall, 1961), p. 24.

2. Henri J. M. Nouwen, *Reaching Out* (Garden City, N. Y.: Doubleday, 1975), p. 54.

3. Ibid., p. 51.

10

The Voices on Cancer Care: A Lens Unfocused and Narrowed

ALDEN SPROULL

Cancer is a disease that has deep spiritual, emotional, and cultural implications. For most people in our society the diagnosis of cancer is a death sentence. Many are even concerned about its "contagiousness." It is perceived as dirty and invasive, ravaging the body and distorting the spirit. It is a disease that induces guilt ("My vaginal cancer came from that affair thirty years ago"), that arouses fear ("I know I am dying, but will it be painful?"), that provokes doubt ("Can I really believe the CT-scan?").

Cancer is an insidious, slowly progressive disease. The course is crisis ridden, its jogs and turns are sudden, and its effects are visible.

I am a photographer by avocation. Photographic concepts help me to understand the reactions to cancer. Just as a photographer utilizes various lenses to capture that special picture, I have found that cancer patients during the course of their disease utilize different lenses for clarity or sharpness or blurredness.

Prior to cancer most people can be perceived as looking through a normal lens, with fairly broad vision and clarity of perspective. With the diagnosis of cancer, the lens becomes unfocused and scattered; everything appears jumbled and cluttered. Once treatment has been started and the cancer comes under control, there is a renewed sense of clarity but with a narrower focus. Recurrence of the disease knocks the picture out of focus. If one reaches the terminal phase of cancer, the focus is close-up, peripheral vision is blurred, and only the most valued things of life are clear.

This illustration is not to suggest a rigidly defined process of stages in cancer. Rather, it is intended to suggest a process that is flexible and changeable, much like a photographic lens.

Pre-Cancer: Vision Wide, Broad, and Clear

We live our lives as though nothing serious is ever going to happen to us, assuming that this life is ours to hold and to keep. The diagnosis of cancer shatters this illusion. Suddenly we are confronted by the uncertainty and finiteness of life.

Yet we who minister to people whose lives have been changed by cancer may still be harboring illusions about our own lives that separate us from the world of the cancer patient. Hence, we have much to learn from cancer patients. In listening to them we discover a variety of coping resources that range broadly in effectiveness. From things they have said, I have been immensely helped in my ministry to them.

The following are taken from comments some cancer patients have shared.

Don't expect too much from us around the time of diagnosis, recurrence, or admission for treatments — we have all we can do just to survive.

Remember we as a family have developed ways to respond to crises in the past, and that we will use them. Good or bad, this is what we bring to the present problem. Don't judge our family or me too severely.

Many of us feel some sense of responsibility for our illness. We know it's illogical, but we still feel it. Don't try too soon to talk us out of it.

We do know clearly what we need or want from you. We know you are a pastor and at times that gets in the way because it reminds us that we are dying. Sometimes we want to escape you, just as sometimes we want to escape the reality of our situation.

What we do want is for you to be a friend, at times a counselor, at times our intercessor-communicator with God. Don't try too hard to do too much for us.

We bring our own unique religious history. We expect you to respect that uniqueness, yet we want you to challenge us at appropriate times to grow beyond our moorings.

Don't talk down to us. Don't make us feel lousy that we're sick. We need for you to treat us normally even though we may be dying.

That's expecting much, but we've come to expect much from ourselves and others.

Be flexible, do not treat us just as another cancer patient. We are
unique persons with unique needs, we want our individuality to be
respected so that we can retain our unique identity as long as possible.

These reflections have taught me much about cancer, and those who
have the disease. They have also informed my ministry. They have suggested that my ministry be flexible, sometimes supportive, other times
confrontational; and individualized, respecting the unique needs and
varying moods of each cancer patient.

Cancer Detection: The Picture Is Jumbled

Irene was forty-three years of age. Several months earlier she had
been diagnosed with pancreatic cancer. She reported to me that her life
had fallen apart due to the cancer. She had become demanding of
everyone. This included a demand that she be told "the truth and nothing but the truth."

After several heated conversations with Irene's oncologist, he finally
spelled out the issues clearly. She became so enraged that she fired her
physician and hired one who would support her viewpoints. Obviously
she was confused and ambivalent. She could not handle the truth which
she demanded. She needed some of her denial supported. The demands
she placed upon her family and others were her need for them to be close
to her in her crisis. Yet the demands were driving them further from
her. The diagnosis of cancer had been devastating for her. The whole
picture was blurred and out of focus, as was her behavior.

Peter was in his late sixties when he was diagnosed with lung cancer.
Upon entering Peter's room, he threw up his hands and declared that he
had nothing to say, that he did not want or desire any "clergy-types"
around. Yet the staff and family reported numerous religious concerns
that he had identified in speaking with them. Sensing the ambivalence,
I finally proposed that I visit with him daily but would only discuss religion at his initiative. Cautiously, he agreed to my proposed contract.

Others experience this "jumbled picture" on a limited scale. They
find it necessary to move toward a focus of clarity for support and coping. Mary, twenty-four, was a special-education instructor. Diagnosed
with acute leukemia, she was very hopeful that aggressive treatments

would effect a remission and enable her to return to teaching. She read voraciously about her disease and came to know almost as much about it as her doctor. Details of the disease became an obsession. Many other activities were suspended. It was her way of coping, but it also threw life out of focus for her.

For still others, the focus remains uncluttered. Pamela, seven years of age, was diagnosed with a cancerous brain tumor. The words of Scripture, "and a little child shall lead them," often came to mind as we talked together. After the initial surgery and radiation, Pam expressed few fears about anything. She continued to live her life to the fullest. I remember a very special gift that she gave me. She had memorized Paul's description of Love (agape) from 1 Corinthians 13. It was a very moving experience. She demonstrated complete trust and faith in a God whom she loved and believed would take care of her. She talked about heaven and her excitement about someday being there. She periodically talked about the sadness that she felt at leaving her family. But wherever she was in her illness, she responded with renewed hope and courage.

Pamela did not have many of life's entrapments to hold her back. She faced each day with the simplicity of a child. Life remained in focus for Pam. The picture was unblurred. Pamela had a very special faith. It was unique and all of those around her were challenged by it.

From these vignettes one can see that ministry to cancer patients can be demanding and exhausting, as the disease is to the patient. In such a ministry I have found that listening is extremely important. What are the unique meanings and needs of the individual? What is the person's story? How is this person coping? What coping resources are there within and beyond this person? How can I intersect this person's life in a meaningful way? Am I able to become a caring participant in his or her rage, tears, sorrow, guilt, and grief? Can I be fully available to cancer patients as they confront life's boundaries? Can I stay with them when the lens becomes jumbled and chaotic?

Cancer under Control: Renewed Clarity

As the incidence of cancer increases, so do the fears and myths deepen. As the incidence of cancer increases, so do the treatment modalities. Treatment often effects remission of varying lengths of times. When remission occurs, it usually induces hope mingled with apprehension. One asks if it is for real or how long it will last or can it be trusted.

It is during this time that hope is reevaluated. Everything in life is based on some level of hope. A cancer patient's hope has a variety of levels. Hope for a cure. Hope for more time. Hope for relief from suffering. Hope that one can still accomplish some personal goals. Often patients in remission will resume the tasks of life with renewed vigor. It almost suggests that if one can busily engage the tasks of life then one is well. Vigorous activity is associated with health.

However, at the same time, many cancer patients in remission approach those tasks with a new perspective. It is rare that one can push against the boundaries of life and not be deeply affected. Some alter their life's goals. Some experience a serenity that comes from a reappraisal of values and goals. Many feel they are living on borrowed time and savor the moments and experiences as they come. Some push down on the accelerator and feverishly seek to accomplish in months or years what they had expected to accomplish in a lifetime.

For many cancer patients the deeper meanings in life are more sharply focused even though the course of their disease remains undetermined. *It is indeed a beautiful irony to feel inner serenity and composure while one's external life is fraught with uncertainty.*

Cancer Recurs: The Focus Is Jumbled and Narrowed

Recurrence of cancer is a devastating experience. It shatters one's confidence in treatment; it actualizes one's worst fears. Many of the feelings encountered in the detection phase resurface, sometimes with even more intensity. It means the disease is out of control. It means life for that person is out of control.

Irene grew worse as time went on and her care became so complex that her family came to the realization that she could not be taken care of at home. There was one major difficulty: Irene had made her family promise that she would not have to return to the hospital.

When she was readmitted to the hospital by her family (against her wishes), she felt betrayed. I entered her room shortly after admission and found her sullen, resentful, and detached. Not only did she feel betrayed by her family, who went against her wishes, but also by God, who did not maintain her remission. She felt helpless, at the mercy of a family that made arbitrary decisions against her will, at the mercy of a disease, now out of control, at the mercy of a capricious God she could no longer trust. Irene's focus had become jumbled and confused and I sought to share in Irene's hurt and rage. She was able to see her family's helplessness. She was able to forgive her father and husband. Irene died unable to "forgive" God who, in her opinion, had betrayed her.

Mary returned to the hospital six months after discharge, out of remission and in need of additional chemotherapy. Bill, her husband, had great difficulty accepting Mary's illness. Mary sensed this and withdrew from Bill. She turned instead to her mother, who became the primary caregiver. In her regression Mary drew closer to her mother as she distanced herself from her husband. Mary struggled with these issues; but the experience was too difficult to handle without mother. The focus was jumbled.

During this recurrence phase it is very difficult for the professional to fully empathize with the cancer patient. There is a chasm that is difficult to span. It is difficult, at times, to accept the regression, the rage, the cynicism, the fear, and futility that are often expressed.

Difficult though it may be, it is extremely important that those ministering to cancer patients be secure in accepting their own limits and finiteness. This is not easy to do when one's own life is filled with buoyancy, energy, and power. *The wide contrast in mood, outlook, and situation in life between cancer and noncancer persons can make communication between them strained.* For a hospital chaplain, filled with vitality and a zest for life, to enter into the deep anguish of one whose life is rapidly ebbing is indeed a demanding challenge.

Dying: Vision Narrowed and Sharpened

It is often in dying that our focus upon living is sharpened. Such persons begin to obliterate the peripheral and extraneous and to concentrate upon that which is vital and important.

Peter was in and out of the hospital several times in the last six months of his life. I visited him regularly and participated in staffings with him, but conformed to the contract that I never initiate any discussion of religion. So did he.

During Peter's last admission, he called me to his room; Ruth, his wife, was in tears. They both knew that he was dying. Ruth had difficulty in saying goodbye. Peter was gasping for air. He looked at me and with great difficulty, thanked me for keeping my end of the contract but now asked that I pray with him. He struggled to share some feelings about his relationship with the church. We held hands together, prayed and asked God to be present with both Peter and Ruth. His words at the conclusion of the prayer spoke of peace and rest. The lens was sharpened. In a short fifteen minutes Peter died.

Jane is a new patient. She knows that she has only weeks to live. This knowledge is enabling her to accept the painful realities of her life. "I postponed having a child for my teaching career. I will never be able to teach those children again. Now the most important aspect of my life is my husband and family. Whatever time I have left I will use that time to experience them and to prepare all of us for my dying."

Many patients begin a process of purging and refining which is common. How they do it, and where they now focus their energies, will vary. My task as a chaplain is to support the process: *to help them withdraw from that which once consumed their life powers and to focus their energies upon that which is most vital to them now.* This ministry helps such persons to sift and refine their basic values.

It is a process that is fraught with religious dimensions. It is a process all persons ought to engage but few actually do. The cancer patient, now confronted with a life-terminating disease, is virtually compelled by that situation to a narrow and sharpened focus. Such a person no longer has the time or the stamina to dissipate energies in a vast array of activities.

Such are the potential losses and gains in one who is dying of cancer: as one is surrendering life, living may take on a deeper and sharper focus.

Pastoral Care to Cancer Patients

In ministering to cancer patients I find that my initial task is to understand how the individual perceives that crisis. There is a direct relationship between perception and coping. What does it mean for this person to have cancer? What is being threatened? What are the significant losses? Only the patient can tell us. My role is to listen and discern.

Then I want to know the coping capacities of this individual. What are the strengths and resources? How can they be effectively mobilized? How has this person habitually coped with similar losses? Can those coping mechanisms be made useful now? Who are the significant people in this person's life? What role are they able to play now?

Finally, I want to help this person to respond in as meaningful, responsible, and creative way as possible. This includes helping the cancer patient to identify and assess options. What choices does this person have, now and in the near future? What are the consequences of either pursuing or ignoring those choices? In what way are one's basic values expressed through those choices? Only the individual can make those decisions. My role is to facilitate that process and to support the individual's capacity and right to choose.

Some of the decisions may have to do with the continuation or modification of treatment. Others have to do with job, family, initiating life-style changes, making provisions for one's possible death. Some have to do with the intense emotions that often surge to the surface. Others have to do with one's relationship to God. Some have to do with the *past*, with regrets and unfulfilled dreams; some with the *present*, with acceptance and adjustment; some with *future* plans and provisions for self and others. I find that my ministry attempts to weave its way through a maze of dynamics, problems, variables, and decisions that are complex and demanding.

Not to be overlooked is the cancer patient's family which is being confronted by severe change and potential loss. The family's internal structure of relationships can help and/or hinder this process. As individuals vary, so do families. Some will communicate openly about the situation, others will be more guarded. Some will overindulge the patient in possessive and protective ways. Some will withdraw their emotional investment. Some will be able to deal directly and responsibly about decisions and tasks. Others will need to deny the realistic implications of the cancer.

This much can be said without qualification: *both patient and loved ones are going through an upheaval; both are facing losses; both may need to make significant changes in their living patterns; both need support to help them deal with each other and with themselves.*

In my ministry to cancer patients I observe many dichotomies. Some patients are at peace with the satisfaction that theirs has been a rich and full life; others are filled with remorse because too much has been left undone. Some want to die because life under present conditions offers no hope for the future; while others lack desire to live because their life has been fraught with failure. Some express a firm belief in eternity yet cling tenaciously to this life; others express no such hope yet die serenely. Some feel closer to God in their dying, while others feel distance. Some willingly relinquish control and place their fate in the hands of others, while others press for more information and fear the growing loss of control. As people are different in living, so they are no less different in dying.

An important part of my ministry is to help cancer patients and families to realize that their intense emotions are appropriate vehicles of communication. The everyday experiences of living with cancer can cause revolt, resentment, hatred, rage, bitterness. Since these are real, authentic feelings, they are viable means of communication with God and their loved ones. Indeed, they are as useful as feelings of affection. If such intense feelings are denied expression, it is difficult to see how the more positive feelings can be authentically expressed. For we can hardly be ourselves unless we make these feelings known to each other.

If we cannot be open about such feelings to God and to those who love us, then to whom can we be open?

Much growth and intimacy can occur when these honest, though negative, emotions are allowed expression. Once expressed, these often open the door for the warm, affectionate feelings to be expressed.

A cancer diagnosis draws people to the basic issues of life, to the core questions of existence. But they are questions that bring us back to our roots and to our connections.

The chaplain brings a symbolic and personal presence to this quest for the basic issues of life. Through this presence the chaplain tries to meet some of the obvious needs for respect, love, appreciation, listening, and hope. The chaplain seeks to provide a constancy to the shifts and changes in mood and condition.

To minister to those afflicted by cancer is a humbling experience. To walk with those who will soon die and be separated from us, from this life as we know it, is both demanding and draining, both awesome and painful. Such a ministry can impact the values and deepen the spirituality of the one who ministers. Through such experience the human struggle becomes more vivid. Indeed, those who minister become co-sojourners in the most intimate, challenging experiences of life.

11

The Voices on Coronary Care:
A Confrontation with Vulnerability

ROBERT STROMBERG

Listening to the voices of vulnerability is the chaplain's function on coronary care. Ministering to coronary patients provides a rich opportunity to encounter some of the most challenging issues of life. Because the heart is viewed as the sustainer of life, any threat to that vital organ threatens life's very existence. It is a threatening and challenging experience for heart patients to face their own mortality, to reevaluate life-long priorities and to make significant life-style changes.

The role of the chaplain in ministering to individuals facing this crisis is threefold: (1) to be an empathetic listener; (2) to be a confronter of reality; and (3) to be a fellow pilgrim who can help articulate the meaning of the inner journey.

The chaplain's first role is *to be an empathetic listener*. Meaningful relationships begin with the recognition that one is being listened to and understood. The patient's relationships begin with the physician and nursing staff, into whose hands the patient's life is entrusted. The primary focus of these medical personnel is on the physical assessment and the development of a treatment plan. But patients often value the presence of a nonmedical person who can focus upon their emotional and spiritual responses to such a life-threatening crisis. The chaplain has the opportunity to bring that presence. While patients use the chaplain as a sounding board to deal with medical questions and concerns they are reluctant to raise with the medical personnel, the chaplain's primary function is to listen to the deeply personal concerns that surface during the illness. Compared to the technology of the coronary care unit, listening may appear insignificant, but it provides a meaningful contribution to the healing process.

The second role of the chaplain is to be a *confronter of reality*. The reality of heart disease and hospitalization may be enough to confront most individuals with their vulnerability, but some may require the assistance of physicians, family, and chaplain. The chaplain may be particularly helpful in enabling patients to face the reality of their mortality and the implications that this has on their life-style. The most effective confrontation avoids a judgmental attitude and conveys the care and understanding of a fellow pilgrim. Confrontation may be a painful experience for those coronary patients who realize their life-style has contributed to their illness. Yet, it is a necessary confrontation if healing is to occur.

The most unique role of the chaplain is to be an *articulator of the inner journey of the coronary patient*. Hospitalization allows the time for reflection. A sensitive chaplain can facilitate and guide such reflection. Many questions surface, questions of one's fragility, of God's role, of personal limitations and responsibilities, of priorities and values. The answer to these and other questions will have a profound effect on the healing process of the heart patient.

Prehospitalization: The Warning of Vulnerability

Symptoms that suggest heart disease vary. They may include pain in the chest, back, or arms, shortness of breath, nausea, weakness, perspiration, or rapid heart rate. The symptoms vary in intensity and frequency and may be brought on by physical activity or emotional stress. They may occur while one is completely at rest. There is no typical set of symptoms that clearly suggest heart disease. Since these symptoms are related to many other illnesses, self-diagnosis is difficult.

People's response to such symptoms also vary. The most typical response is denial: to assume they're not serious and will go away; or to conclude that the symptoms suggest indigestion or the flu. It is common to hide symptoms from others, especially those significant others who would become alarmed and recommend immediate medical attention. The denial of symptoms has little to do with educational background. According to Dr. Thomas P. Hackett, a psychiatrist who has worked extensively with heart patients at Massachusetts General Hospital, it is the typical response to a life-threatening crisis. He asserts that physicians and particularly cardiologists, are no different from the rest of the population in needing to deny symptoms. He relates a story of a well-known cardiologist who, while speaking on the topic of heart disease, experienced the symptoms of a heart attack, but insisted that he had merely choked on a fish bone. Even after he was told he was having a heart attack, he could not accept this reality until he could do his own electrocardiogram.

The need to deny the possibility of a life-threatening illness is a common human response. However, when physical symptoms become so intense that they cannot be ignored, or when significant others become aware of the symptoms, medical assistance is sought, which usually means a visit to a hospital emergency room for an evaluation. Often the decision to seek medical assistance is made by a family member, who is better able to make an objective assessment. Many lives are saved by what are called "executive wives," who are willing to make such decisions over the protests of their husbands.

With heart disease time is crucial. Most deaths occur because of the delay in receiving adequate medical attention. The great majority of people who reach the hospital survive their attack.

Hospitalization: Confrontation with Vulnerability

The patient's denial of symptoms is immediately challenged by the hospital's environment. The drama and excitement that accompany the involvement of the paramedics, with their initial assessment and treatment, challenge the notion that all is well. Any patient brought into the emergency room with chest pains or other suspicious symptoms receives the urgent attention of the staff. This clearly signals crisis. It now becomes more difficult to deny the seriousness of the symptoms. While arrival in a hospital emergency room may increase the level of anxiety, it may also decrease that level. The knowledge that one is being attached to a heart monitor, being assessed by expert medical staff, and being given medications may be reassuring to one who feels in danger. If the evidence suggests the slightest suspicion of heart pathology, the patient is admitted to a coronary unit for further evaluation.

The period of testing and evaluating may be a time of considerable anxiety. The unknowns at this stage in hospitalization may allow people to continue their denial or to fantasize the most serious types of illness. Not knowing the truth about one's condition is a troublesome dilemma. Living with such unknowns is a challenge to one's faith in God and one's trust in others.

Response to Diagnosis

Like the originating symptoms, the response to any diagnosis may be disbelief. While people naturally resist dealing with their own vulner-

ability, *it is the most significant issue that confronts coronary patients.*
How a person deals with this spiritual issue affects the way in which
other issues are dealt with during rehabilitation. For until a person accepts the reality of his or her mortality, there will be little motivation for
making any significant life-style changes which are vital in prolonging
life. It is with this issue that the chaplain may make the most unique and
significant contribution to the coronary patient.

When the reality of the illness breaks through disbelief, people begin
to respond more realistically. In his book *The Cardiac Patient*,[1] Dr.
George Patterson, a hospital chaplain, describes the varied responses to
life-threatenting illness. He suggests a variety of responses that don't fit
any sequential pattern or progressive movement.

Denial

Denial is a normal and healthy defense against the possibility of immi-
nent danger or death. It is a helpful coping mechanism that enables one
to gather the resourses necessary to address the crisis. There is evidence
that people who have healthy denial systems are better survivors in
crises. The ability to deny the possible imminence of death prevents the
flood of emotions that can easily overwhelm the victim, adversely affecting judgment and decision making. An overwhelming flood of emotions
may create a physiological response in the body in which catecholamines
(hormones) are released into the blood system thereby enhancing its
clotting efficiency. While this may be helpful to a person in an accident
or under attack from an enemy, it can threaten the life of coronary patients whose arteries are already narrowed by atherosclerosis. It is therefore important to respect this defense of denial until the person is ready
to deal more fully with the reality of the situation.

However, denial can be an unhealthy response if it prevents a person
from eventually dealing with the seriousness of the crisis. When denial
persists, it may lead to dangerous overactivity and a lack of responsibility
for one's own health care. Such denial that persists needs to be confronted
and challenged.

Fear and Anxiety

Fear may have many sources: pain, being a burden to others, death.
Fear may be determined by the circumstances surrounding hospitalization, severity of symptoms, personality, and past experiences of the patient.

Once in the hospital the patient's fear may be variously focused, for example, on the diagnostic and therapeutic activities, the effects of hospitalization on one's family and job. Fearful questions emerge concerning one's future capabilities. In such cases the greatest expressed fear of the patient is not of dying, but the fear of being an invalid.

Similar but different is anxiety, a vague undefined fear of the unknown. It is apprehension that has no specific focus. Anxiety may be expressed through nervous talking, asking numerous questions, or an inability to concentrate. Anxiety is difficult to deal with because of its unknown source. The better able a person is to identify its sources, the less anxious that person is likely to be.

Anger, Shame, and Guilt

Another response to life-threatening illness and the enforced restrictions of hospitalization is anger. While it is a normal expression of discontent and dissatisfaction, anger is seldom overtly expressed, in part because its expression is seen as the inappropriate loss of control. For some religious people anger is seen as a lack of faith. The inability to express such a normal emotion as anger may contribute to confusion and/or depression.

But toward whom can anger be expressed? Toward God? That may be impossible for people who believe that God has spared their life. Toward their physicians? The nurses? Occasionally, but because of one's dependency upon their skills and care, the patient is hesitant to incur their wrath. Toward family? Sometimes, because their sustained loyalty is assumed. But in this predicament the coronary patient may fear even their abandonment. The anger may also be focused on the dietary and physical restrictions necessitated by the illness.

Shame is the sense of being embarrassed. Illness impairs one's productivity. It suggests idleness and weakness and dependency. Since self-esteem is related to self-reliance and independence, their loss can arouse shame or embarrassment. Shame may adversely affect the patient's relationship to those who seek to help, for to be helped suggests vulnerability. (This may be a reason some church members do not notify their pastors and congregations when they are hospitalized.)

A more expected response is guilt. Questions may be asked like: why did this happen to me? Am I being punished? Is God trying to say something to me? Such questions imply cause and effect and retribution. Many people suffer from "neurotic guilt" that is related to unrealistic goals and expectations that can never be met, resulting in feelings of failure and guilt.

Heart patients need to deal with some real guilt when they learn that their life-style has contributed to their heart disease. Patients will be reminded that smoking cigarettes, poor nutritional habits, lack of regular exercise, uncontrolled blood pressure and diabetes, and stressful life-styles may have contributed to their heart disease. Accepting responsibility for the consequences of those "sins" may be a painful but redemptive experience. Chaplains can be helpful in differentiating between real guilt, which is related to abuse and overindulgence, and neurotic guilt, which is related to perfectionism and unhealthy competition.

Depersonalization, Isolation, and Loneliness

Being hospitalized is a depersonalizing experience. The needs of an efficiently operated hospital require a certain amount of conformity that negates personal tastes and freedom. The focus upon the physical and medical aspects of a person's life may inadvertently devalue many uniquely personal qualities. The life-saving technology of a critical-care unit itself can have a depersonalizing effect on the patient and family.

Illness of any kind isolates the ill person from the normal healthy population. Patients, for the most part, are isolated from their families, friends, work, and meaningful activities. And while some of those relationships are maintained, the context of the hospital makes them different. The nature of a critical illness may cause people to look inward rather than outward for meaning. Such introspection may provide people with a rare opportunity to wrestle with the meaning of their life and with the quality of their relationships with God, family, and significant others. But such introspection can induce loneliness.

Emptiness and Depression

When a person's self-image is assaulted by the losses of illness, emptiness results. Those whose identity has been molded by being active and productive may feel diminished, with nothing significant to contribute. The heart patient experiences many losses, some of which will be temporary, that is, dignity, work, family involvement, certainty. Depression is a common reaction to loss.

The symptoms of depression include feelings of worthlessness, self-doubt, a lack of energy and an inability to concentrate. The usual mechanisms for coping with depression (e.g., investment in meaningful work or activity, exercise, or travel) are not available to heart patients during their convalescence. They seriously wonder if such activities will ever be available to them again.

Posthospitalization: Coping with Vulnerability

Reflecting on the crisis of a life-threatening disease can be a difficult but meaningful experience. Becoming aware of the reality of one's mortality can give rise to the opportunity for growth and healing. Out of physical, emotional, and spiritual pain, a person can gain a new perspective on the meaning of life. In order for such growth to occur, there needs to be a motivation for growth, an accepting environment in which growth can occur, and available people who are willing to engage patients in their struggle with issues.

The Issue of Identity: Who Am I?

For the heart patient who has faced a life-threatening experience, there may come a new understanding of the self as truly mortal. Will it happen again? Will help be available? Will my activities contribute to another attack? All are questions that reflect that new understanding. The intensity of these concerns will decrease in time, but to some degree will always influence the way in which people view themselves.

Patients' views of themselves go through a number of stages following their attack. Initially, heart patients see themselves as "fragile survivors," susceptible to further attacks. In time, patients will go through a period of "ambiguity and conflict," a time of confusion and uncertainty about future roles and personal competence. This is followed by a period in which patients see themselves as "normal, but different." Finally, heart patients see themselves as people who have had an attack and are now living new lives with a fuller awareness of boundaries and limits. In giving up notions of immortality, patients must also surrender notions of omnipotence which claims the power to accomplish any and all goals.

The Challenge of Life-Style Change: What Can I Still Do?

The prognosis for most heart patients is good. A part of the optimism is related to the fact that people can minimize or eliminate a number of risk factors that may have contributed to their disease. The challenge of making life-style changes is one of the most difficult issues facing the coronary patient. Patients are asked to change meaningful habits that have been established over a lifetime. This requires a major effort. Sometimes people are challenged to change three or four risk factors at the same time. The patient may well wonder whether any activity is free from harm. The most difficult challenge facing the coronary patient, however, is the need to change personality traits that may have been responsible for their career success (i.e., driving competitiveness, perfectionism).

Undoubtedly, the family will play a significant role in helping the patient make those life-style changes deemed necessary. Because of their emotional involvement, family members may focus their attention on the patient's *need* to change rather than the *struggle* that is involved in making such changes. While support to change is needed, heart patients will also need to be with others who will understand and appreciate the struggles involved in such changes.

The Response of Family: Will They Still Love Me?

Families are deeply affected by a life-threatening crisis. Will the patient live? How long will the patient live? These and more are questions that are raised during the crisis and remain for a long time. As families entrust their loved ones to the care of professionals, who they may know only by reputation, they experience feelings of "helplessness" and "isolation." It is ironic that during the critical phase of heart disease the most significant people in the patient's life are the least involved and the most isolated.

While it is appropriate that the patient's needs be the primary focus of the hospital staff, family needs often go unaddressed. Consequently, families often feel uninformed and ill prepared to provide the appropriate care when the patient returns home. An important function of the chaplain is to provide a needed link between the family and the medical staff.

During the rehabilitation stage there may be a temporary reversal of roles, which adds stress for both the patient and family. It is particularly difficult for men to sit back and watch their wives undertake physical tasks formerly assumed by them. For the person whose self-image has already been injured, this may be a highly sensitive issue.

When the patient is released from the hospital to the care of the family, there may be a loss of security that came through the hospital's care. To shift that care to the family can create anxiety. If the family views the heart patient as a fragile person who needs constant monitoring, they will be anxious and become overprotective. While the overprotection is normal and needs to be understood as the family's way of expressing concern, it can create stress for the patient. One patient interpreted the family's overprotection as an indication that he was much sicker than had been indicated to him by his doctors.

It is unfortunate that at the time when the family is trying to gain more control by giving care, the patient is endeavoring to assume more self-control. The conflict that evolves from these mixed expectations will need to be understood and addressed.

Sexual Relationships: How Can I Express My Love?

Following the crisis of a life-threatening illness, couples may have a need for more affection and intimacy. This may create some stress since the heart patient may not participate in sexual intercourse for a period of time. When sexual activity is resumed, couples will need to deal with questions of its safety for and its effect upon the heart patient, as well as the best/safest conditions for sexual activity.

Since sexual activity is a much neglected topic among medical personnel, couples will need to be encouraged to initiate discussion with their physician regarding their personal questions. Couples also need to communicate with each other their desires, fears, and expectations regarding this significant area of life. While there is usually no medical reason why couples cannot resume their normal level of sexual activity, there may be a diminished interest because of heart medications or depression.

Conflict over Nutrition: What Can I Eat?

Diet may be an issue which creates conflict between patient and family. Since a number of risk factors for heart disease are related to nutrition, the family (and especially the wife) may feel guilty about nutritional practices that could have contributed to the heart disease. They may now become overly zealous about monitoring the patient's diet. While patients may welcome the concern, they may not appreciate the control that others assume in restricting their diet. Heart patients need to take responsibility for their own lives. This is an area which requires the understanding and cooperation of the whole family.

The Significance of Work: Will I Be Productive Again?

One of the chief concerns of employed coronary patients is the prospect of returning to work. They may wonder if there is still a job, since heart disease is a liability for some types of work (people in the construction and transportation industry may no longer be employable at their same jobs). While the majority of heart patients return to their same positions, there may be fear that their employer will find other reasons to transfer them to less responsible jobs or to terminate them. For those who are interested in upward mobility, there may be no opportunity for promotions.

Many patients struggle with whether they will be *able* and *willing* to maintain the same high performance standards. This is true especially if patients believe such attitudes, expectations, and values contributed to their illness. They may question whether they want to go back to the same job or, when back on the job, if they will be able to change attitudes and expectations.

One of the ways in which the heart patient may regain self-esteem is by returning to work. Being a productive and contributing member of society is one of the ways in which self-worth is achieved. But returning to work will not be without anxiety as the patient struggles with the need to work and the fear of functioning inadequately. Feelings of depression can distort one's self-image and cause questions and doubt regarding the ability to perform. Fellow employees and employers will welcome back the heart patient, but probably not understand the inner struggles. If the returning employee receives any special treatment (i.e., a shortened work day, a lighter load, or any special consideration), it may give rise to some friendly, or not so friendly, remarks about special hours or about what some people will do to get out of work. From all appearances the coronary patient looks like the "picture of health," therefore any preferential treatment will appear inappropriate. This issue places an additional burden upon the returning heart patient.

Although most people return to their same employment, they will probably approach work differently. The crisis of surviving a life-threatening illness raises some spiritual issues regarding the meaning of work. Is self-worth attained by productivity? What is the value of work—a means to financial security, a means of self-fulfillment, or a means of service to others? The struggle with these questions often results in some creative work changes, that is, delegating more responsibility, adopting less competitive attitudes, and being more realistic about expectations.

The Response of Friends: Will They Stand by Me?

The care and support of friends during a crisis can be a meaningful and humbling experience, especially to those who may not have appreciated the value of such relationships. In many instances those friendships will be more highly valued. Friends can also be a source of disappointment when they do not provide the support expected. Some friends may see their own vulnerability in the heart patient and avoid him or her. What happened suddenly to the victim of a heart attack may happen to them.

Attitudes toward Medications:
Do I Need to Depend on Medications?

Medications play an important role in contributing to the health of the coronary patient. These agents of God's healing may regulate blood pressure, heart rate, heart rhythm, or serve as anticoagulants. Patients are taught the purpose and value of these medications. Some patients see these as life-saving drugs and will take their medications regularly. Other patients see medications as a reminder of their weakness and are therefore eager to be free of medication. Once again, the heart patient's honest willingness to confront the realities of one's mortality is an important factor.

Ambivalence about Going Home:
Am I Well Enough to Leave the Hospital?

The most often asked question in the hospital is when can one go home. The usual response is to wait and see how things go. While this is a necessary physician response, it leaves the patient with some anxiety. When the discharge day is near, the physician may say that the patient can go tomorrow if everything looks good or if the patient's test allows it. Such cautious responses remind patients of the precariousness of their situation. When the discharge day arrives, patients may experience anxiety about leaving the protective environment of the hospital where medical care is minutes away. This is coupled with an eagerness to return to familiar surroundings and to regain some control over their life.

The Meaning of Pain: Will I Have Another Heart Attack?

For the person who has had a heart attack, or open heart surgery, pain is a very sensitive issue. The slightest pain or discomfort in the chest becomes a signal for concern. This sensitivity will diminish as time and experience teach that all pain and discomfort are not related to heart disease. However, since pain is a symptom that should be taken seriously, coronary patients will need to learn how to evaluate their pain and to know when medical help should be sought.

Resources for Coping with Vulnerability

The experience of a life-threatening illness creates a spiritual crisis in the life of the coronary patient. Survival of the crisis is often followed by a period of reflection. It is often a time of struggling with life's beliefs, values, and goals. For some, heart disease may be seen as punishment, justly or unjustly deserved. For others, heart disease may be seen as a reprieve—an opportunity to make a new beginning. And for still others, it will be seen as an opportunity for growth and spiritual healing.

For most people, surviving such an illness results in an overwhelming sense of gratitude to God. This gratitude may be expressed overtly through words of gratitude, prayer, or acts of worship; or covertly, through attitudes of appreciation, love, and hope.

Among recovering coronary patients there is a strong sense of well-being and hopefulness. This encouraging outlook is related partially to the medical assurance that most patients will be able to return to a normal life-style. But this hopefulness also grows out of a belief that heart patients can find meaning in life, despite life's limitations. The potential such meaning provides improves the quality of their lives.

Heart disease challenges many of our deeply held assumptions about life. It challenges the belief that humans are indestructable and is a stark reminder that we cannot always trust our bodies. It also challenges our reliance upon position and material wealth. It further challenges our indispensability to work, family, and community.

As these assumptions are being challenged, heart patients can discover the value of trusting others. It begins by literally placing one's life in the hands of physicians and nurses whose skill and knowledge help sustain life. Patients may also learn how trustworthy their family and friends may be in time of crisis.

Trust in God is the ultimate evidence of a growing faith. With the growing awareness of what is tangible and not worthy of trust, what is immortal and worthy of trust becomes more apparent. When everything in life seems to be falling apart, God is experienced as the one who is dependable and who can give meaning and value to life. God's love enables some heart patients to accept themselves despite their unhealthy life-style and their misplaced priorities.

Having experienced the meaning of being loved in a deeper way, many heart patients are better able to offer love to others, to be more compassionate toward those facing similar boundaries. Many patients, in response to their experience, are eager to give to others what they have received—love.

NOTES

1. George Patterson, *The Cardiac Patient* (Minneapolis: Augsburg Publishing House, 1978), pp. 98-105.

12

The Voices of the Dying
and the Bereaved:
A Bridge Between Loss and Growth

LEROY B. JOESTEN

How does someone help another person die? How does someone help another person "let go" of a loved one who has died? Chaplains are certainly not the only professionals who must wrestle with these questions. Nor are we to assume that times of death or grief are the only times chaplains can be useful. But chaplains are selected by many to help them deal with dying and grieving. Chaplains are expected to know something about life beyond death and how we may ready ourselves for what lies beyond the grave. Chaplains are expected to know something about life's meaning, its purpose and direction.

Helping people die or grieve, however, is based less on "knowing" and more on "believing." And even more than believing, the ability to help is based on how well we have integrated into our own lives what we believe to be true, not only about death but also about life. This chapter attempts to identify the basic human reactions to death and grief and to demonstrate how the chaplain's integration of life and death themes becomes the foundation for ministering to the dying and bereaved.

Ministering to the Dying

Even though all can anticipate death, not every death is anticipated. Some people die suddenly and unexpectedly. These individuals are spared the agony of facing their mortality and their loved one's reactions to their eventual death. Most people, however, die with some forewarning. The period of time given to anticipate death challenges these dying persons to come to terms with their own death and to reconcile themselves to their survivors' existence without them.

Given the opportunity to prepare for death, people may react in various ways. Some seek to live life as normally as possible. Little changes in life-style are made, but previous patterns are seized more firmly. Others use the opportunity to number their days, to reevaluate and rearrange priorities. Changes, even drastic, can and do occur. Some dissolve their marriage and others quit their job, while others may demonstrate a new religious fervor. Some diseases are so aggressive they leave the dying little time or physical strength to make changes or even to resume their normal patterns.

Elizabeth Kübler-Ross's well-known and monumental work with the terminally ill gave rise to the so-called five stages of death and dying. These five stages received much criticism because they imply a progressive movement from denial to acceptance and because such stages are difficult to assess. George Fitchett, a chaplain at Rush-Presbyterian St. Luke's, Chicago (in a study entitled "Testing the Validity of Kübler-Ross' Stage Theory," presented at the Fourth Annual Meeting of the National Hospice Organization in 1981), asked 156 health care professionals to evaluate a written patient interview in terms of the five stages. Forty-four percent of the raters judged the patient to be in the state of acceptance, 12 percent judged the patient to be in denial, and 44 percent in some other emotional state. This diversity is noteworthy since the interview had been drawn from Kübler-Ross's book *On Death and Dying*, where it had been used as an illustration of a patient attempting to reach acceptance.[1]

Fitchett appropriately concluded that whereas the stage theory intends to sensitize caregivers, making them more compassionate, it often produces the opposite effect. These categories tempt helpers to stereotype the dying person and tend to oversimplify the process of coming to terms with death. This process can be agonizingly painful and complex for patient, family, and professionals alike.

If we look more closely at the five stages of Kübler-Ross, there really are only two, and they are not states but reactions which remain in dynamic tension, namely, *resistance* and *acceptance*. Denial, anger, bargaining, and depression are merely different expressions of resistance. They are patients' attempts to ward off the necessity of looking at, and dealing with, the inevitability of their death. If we view the stages in this way, we discover that there are different levels of denial and of acceptance. As denial begins to wane, acceptance develops in different degrees. Certain aspects of this process may be accepted, such as the disease and necessary treatments, while other aspects may remain denied, such as the ultimate outcome. Patients require time, energy, and assistance to fully absorb the weight of this total experience.

Rather than trying to move patients through the stages, it is important to recognize that tension between denial and acceptance. Avery Weisman posits this view in his helpful book *On Dying and Denying*.[2] Weisman defines denial as a process. He discusses three orders of denial and acceptance which appear in varying degrees throughout three psychosocial stages of a fatal illness. These stages are primary recognition, established disease, and final decline. First-order denial (denial of the diagnosis) occurs in stage one and early stage two. Second-order denial (denial of the implications of the illness) is common in stage two. Third-order denial (denial of the fatal outcome) is typical during stage three.

This produces three comments regarding denial. First of all, it is a natural emotional response. It keeps the ego from being swept away into oblivion and time from being devalued as having no merit or usefulness.

Second, it is necessary. There must be a degree of denial if a person is to distinguish between the inevitability of death and the imminence of death. (I may know that I am going to die someday, but I am not yet dead.)

Third, those surrounding the dying are caught in a similar tension between being forced by circumstances to surrender the person to death yet being compelled by emotional ties to "hold on" to them. Family members can be heard reminding dying patients how indispensable they are, how life cannot go on without them, and how they must keep fighting. Medical professionals themselves are well known for their resistance to the inevitability or timeliness of certain deaths. Chaplains also can become so attached to some patients that they are deaf to patient overtures to discuss dying.

What is the chaplain's response to this tension between resisting and accepting one's death? I am called to enter into the patient's and family's tension. This requires that chaplains tolerate within themselves the tension between being mortal and being alive. It requires that they not only be familiar with others' views of death but that they have a view of their own death, not for the purpose of superimposing it upon a dying patient, but so it can be a personal reference point in their ministry to those who are dying.

Entering a patient's tension requires a tolerance for sadness. To engage people at all—to learn what moves, excites, frightens, or stimulates them —means we begin to care for them. Whenever we must surrender anyone or anything for which we care, there is pain. Patients who have been receptive to my ministry, who have shared willingly and openly their hopes and fears and have used me to clarify their own feelings about death, have helped me contend with my own dying and the eventual deaths of my loved ones. When those patients die, I am sad because a bond is broken.

Entering this tension requires acceptance of powerlessness. The first major step toward acceptance of death is the admission that we are all powerless to change the *fact* that we will die. Once that hurdle is crossed, we are free to consider the choices we have regarding *when* and *how* to die. *When* we die is certainly determined by behavior, life-styles, eating habits, and the like. William Foege, the Director of the Centers for Disease Control in Atlanta, stated in a 1981 speech: "If you are a part of this group, which feels that you have no control over your destiny, I'd like to make the case that the age of rugged individualism is only now dawning." *How* we die is influenced by our attitudes, beliefs, faith, or how long we will hope that a particular disease can be reversed or prolonged. The husband of a terminally ill woman recently said to his wife and me, "I feel so inadequate, so helpless." His behavior of pushing her to eat, coercing her to walk, and demanding that she come to talk with me reflected a desire to keep her alive. She was resentful of his efforts because she felt they were robbing her of choices involving her living (and her dying).

It is not the chaplain's responsibility to condition a patient's response or to force acceptance. However, acceptance of death is nurtured by bearing witness to death's reality. While I was making a home visit to a young man in his mid-twenties who had lived with cancer for many years, he asked if I thought he looked worse than at the time of my previous visit. As I observed his wasted body, distended stomach, jaundiced complexion, and sunken eyes, I said, "Yes, you do look worse." I was surprised to have him thank me for being honest. He gave me two blank cassettes that he said he would no longer be using. One of his greatest joys was listening to music. He told me they were very good tapes, and he would no longer need them. It was the last time I saw him; he died two days later.

Chaplains are called to bear witness to the truth about death. Whether we choose to face death directly or not, death will not be denied. I frequently ask patients who have a serious illness if they ever think about death. Or I ask them how serious they think their condition is. Such questions give rise to concerns about what they are leaving behind (family, friends, home, unfinished hopes and dreams), as well as what they believe lies ahead.

Not all persons struggle with their dying in the same way. Some by their courage, honesty, and faith are an inspiration in the way they face their death. They help us to number our days. I well remember the woman who spoke a passage from 1 Corinthians 13 as her primary, death-bed hope: "then I shall know, even as I am now known."

People need the freedom to decide what their own response will be toward death, and to some extent, how it will come about (e.g., in physical comfort and clarity of thought or under the rigors of discomforting treatments). Their choices are aided when we give them "permission" to express their feelings, fears, faith, and hopes. My task is to accompany the person who is tossed back and forth between winning and losing, between wanting to fight and wanting to quit. The chaplain symbolizes the reality that discussion of death is not in and of itself negative (as some people believe). On the contrary, to discuss openly one's thoughts, feelings, or questions about death is a positive means of dealing with life's most universal truth. The chaplain walks a fine line between valuing acceptance of death, yet respecting the ego boundaries people set for themselves.

Ministry to the Bereaved

The truth to which chaplains bear witness when ministering to the bereaved is that life does go on without the deceased. In spite of resistance and the bereaved person's protestations, death is not reversible.

The grief experienced by survivors, after a death has occurred, is similar to the grief experienced by the dying person prior to death. The survivors experience the wrenching pain between knowing one set of realities and yet craving another set. In other words, to know is not necessarily to accept. Both the dying and their survivors are required to accept something they don't want to accept. While reality is saying yes, it is happening (in the case of the dying) or it has happened (in the case of the survivors), the person is also saying no. Shock, anger, bargaining are different ways of saying no. There are numerous ways survivors try to "undo" the reality of death. The death seems unfair or untimely or unnecessary. There are so many reasons why a particular event should not be; but it cannot be undone. People can seem tireless in their efforts to undo death. They must be given permission to seek out all these avenues to retrieve the deceased while, at the same time, being reminded gently but firmly of the second truth about death, namely, life does go on. The challenge to come to a point of acceptance necessitates "an emotional

goodbye," a letting go of the deceased, "a sending them away" (This latter phrase was used by Dr. Ronald Ramsey in a dramatic demonstration
of his work with a grieving mother on a segment of the television program
60 Minutes in 1977.).[3]

The process we call grief is the bridge between loss and growth. One
hopes that through that process what was negative will ultimately yield
some potential promise. I discourage even hinting that "something good
will come out of this." Only time and events will tell that for certain. But
it is important for the chaplain to believe that loss and growth do go
hand in hand, and that little growth ever occurs without some accompanying loss or sacrifice.

The tasks of bereavement are twofold: *to disengage or detach*; for the
purpose of *reattaching* or *reinvesting*. One must experience the loss
fully — intellectually, emotionally, physically, and spiritually — in order
to be available to reinvest fully in life.[4]

These tasks have implications for the griever and the chaplain. The
griever is challenged to receive nurture and care from others. Initially,
the bereaved is called upon to be a receiver, to regress to needing in ways
not experienced since childhood. But as the process swings to the side of
reinvesting, the griever must identify, claim, and use those skills, gifts,
and qualities which he or she possesses. There is a time to be helped and
a time to stand on one's own. The challenge for the *chaplain* is to balance the needs to nurture and to encourage; to know when to comfort
and support and when to challenge and confront.

No one can grieve for someone else. But an environment can be established wherein the work of grief can take place. The work of the chaplain
is to allow the bereaved person to grieve and, in time, to allow the bereaved to stop grieving. Initially, experiencing the depths of hurt and pain
is an escape from investing in the life of someone else. Many have said
that grief is the price we pay for loving. But at some point, the bereaved
person must be helped to let go of the crushing pain. This means to realize that there is no relationship which is binding beyond death, and that
to resume one's life fully and joyfully is not a betrayal of or a disservice to
the deceased. Even the promise of faithfulness of a husband and wife is "til
death parts us." In fact, the resumption of one's life and the reinvestment
of one's self can be seen as a tribute and a living memorial to the deceased,
since much of what we are is the result of the other's investment in us.

The Pain of Grief

There perhaps is no better word to describe the experience of grief
than pain. The pain of mourning a loved one is total, sapping one's very

energy. We grieve with our whole being, as we find ourselves fatigued, unable to concentrate, driven by extreme mood swings (temperamental), unappreciative or critical of friends and acquaintances, and often questioning our most basic religious beliefs. Not all losses result in the same level of pain. Circumstances of relationship to the deceased, manner of death, amount of forewarning, personality of the bereaved, and cultural sanctions and prohibitions are all highly influential. Since each set of circumstances can vary, there can be no simple timetable for the duration of pain.

Unlike physical pain, someone in grief must be encouraged to endure the pain, to live with it. It cannot be covered or hidden if it is to be extinguished. This is often the most difficult work for a chaplain, to encourage the arousal of the pain without efforts to erase it. The acute, stabbing pain shortly after a loss usually gives way to a more dull, chronic type of pain as the reality of death makes its way into the bereaved's inner self. The former may be characterized by outward displays of emotion, severe and prolonged episodes of crying; the latter may be characterized by a lack of motivation and of interest in life, general apathy. Both are expressions of pain.

Grief is at one and the same time universal and personal. No matter how much commonality people in grief may experience, the one who is grieving must alone bear the emptiness and separation from one's loved one. Others may try to understand, may be physically present, may be moved to tears, but the utter depths of that loss can never be trivialized by the words, "I know exactly how you feel." I believe many grief stricken people want to feel that they have just experienced the worst tragedy ever experienced by any human being who ever lived. For a time, the greatest comfort comes not in having their pain denied, or belittled, but by demonstrating through our physical presence a willingness to endure with them — as best we can — this devastating experience. (Those who are dependent upon the mourner may not feel the luxury of such endurance.) But life must move on; patience can be tried severely. In time, after the release of the painful feelings, the bereaved themselves begin to put the loss in some kind of overarching perspective, if meaning and purpose are again to emerge in their lives.

The Needs of the Bereaved:
Understanding, Patience, Acceptance

The situation of the bereaved requires *understanding*. Not only is grief painful, but it is interminably painful. The bereaved is on a course which is frighteningly painful and with an uncertain duration. One of the most frequently asked questions is how long will it last. There is the thought that if one knew how long it would last, it could be endured. The difficulty is that it cannot be told in advance, except in very general terms; that is, the acute pain should subside in weeks to a couple months, but the full, aching pain usually lasts eighteen to twenty-four months. The bereaved needs time and reminding that the issue is not merely one of chronology (i.e., the passage of time) but one of readiness, an inner willingness to redirect one's emotional energy from what was, to what is, to what can be (from the past to the present to the future).

One of the ways understanding is conveyed is by listening without judgment, proclamation, or lecture. This can be effectively done by anyone, but is most appreciated when rendered by someone who has experienced a similar loss. Grief support groups are one way of providing such understanding. Understanding is important because the bereaved may be unable to understand themselves and be confused as to what they really want. It is not unusual for those widowed to refuse invitations from long-time friends, because they do not want to go out, and at the same time be angry because friends or neighbors have forgotten them. To say the least, bereavement is a time of confusion and uncertainty. Not only are the bereaved adjusting to new external surroundings and circumstances but also to a new inner person. Somehow they are not the same. Their feelings, attitudes, and temperament are different. Their responses to others are different.

People in grief may seem like strangers to themselves. One reason for this is that they may never before have felt such a wide range of emotions, or at such depth.

Not only is there a new range of thoughts and emotions, but an annoying and disturbing forgetfulness. At one time, our widows' group met in a former parsonage next to a large church in town. The site of our meetings was advertised in a newsletter as being "the house adjacent to the church." One night a well-educated widow who attended the group for the first time embarrassingly confessed in the course of the group, "I had to stop a policeman and ask him what the word *adjacent* meant. I couldn't remember." Bereaved will often say they fear they're going "crazy." They find themselves talking to the deceased, sensing their presence, dreaming about them, and at times convinced they hear their voice. They need reassurance that such experiences are natural and common.

People in grief may be extremely moody, their feelings unpredictable and inconsistent, calling upon all our *patience*. I often describe grief as a full-time profession; the problem is most people cannot afford to work at it full time. There are other demands and responsibilities which they must fulfill. It is not uncommon for a flood of emotion and tears to suddenly erupt. Grateful are those who have sympathetic, patient, and accepting employers and colleagues when these unanticipated outbursts of emotion occur.

A young woman who came frequently to talk with me about the death of her mother conveyed an exchange with a friend who had called her, asking what she might do to help. The young woman declared, "Just be patient with me. Just be patient."

The grieving process cannot be packaged neatly. It is easy for those standing outside of the experience to become impatient with bereaved persons' emotional outbursts, their needs to discuss repeatedly the circumstances of the death, to reminisce and talk about the deceased. That remembering, reminiscing, must be exercised, not as a means to recall the past but to surrender it, to gradually come to the realization that those days are now gone. This encouragement may run counter to the advice of well-meaning others who tell the bereaved to "get your mind off it" and who push the bereaved to sever connections with anything that brings back painful memories.

Patience does not come easily. We are known to be a society in a hurry. We crowd our schedules — days, weeks, months in advance. We overcommit, overextend, and overestimate our ability to handle multiple responsibilities effectively. But when we deal with the dying and the bereaved, time takes on a new dimension.

I am often impressed how impatient the dying and the grieving are with themselves. They are as judgmental of themselves (that they should be stronger or have more faith) as others are of them. They are envious of those people who go through a traumatic event and act and behave as though nothing ever happened. And that is the way we like it. How often does one commend someone who is emotionally distraught or defend a person's right to be upset or angry or frustrated? Recently an advanced cancer patient shared with me her frustration with her family's inability to tolerate her periodic episodes of sadness. She questioned me, "Isn't a person with cancer entitled to some 'down times'?" I assured her she was.

It is at this point that the church and the church's busy schedule betrays its impatience with the bereaved. Many widowed have said that their pastors did not know what to do with them. Couples' clubs no longer seem appropriate because of the fifth-wheel syndrome. Singles' groups frequently mix all ages and all circumstances of singleness (e.g., those who have never been married, those who are divorced, those who are widowed). Whereas this type of social gathering may include all, bereaved individuals have quite distinct needs and deserve separate settings, at least for a time. The issue is that we must alter our schedules and attitudes to accommodate the needs of the dying and bereaved.

Bereavement is a time for *acceptance*, for it can be a time of immense insecurity. It is often a time when one seriously questions one's ability to survive without the deceased. Whereas this is often an unconscious, manipulative ploy to resurrect the deceased, in another sense, it is an expression of that person's inner reservations about one's competence or worthiness to continue living.

Anger can often cause the bereaved to question their worth and value. This anger can erupt in the most gentle of spirits and be directed at friends, professional helpers (i.e., doctors, nurses, clergy), at God (for allowing this death), at the deceased (for abandoning them), or even at one's self (for not having done more to prevent the death). It can take on the tone of jealousy toward other people whose lives go on undisturbed. Widowed individuals will look enviously at older couples who still have a life together. Bereaved parents may harbor feelings of resentment toward parents whose children are healthy, active and vital.

Toward Recovery

How then shall a chaplain help someone who has experienced the sadness and devastation of the death of a loved one? How can the negatives of this loss be converted into an opportunity for growth? The chaplain helps by embodying *someone to hope with them, to believe in them, and to be honest with them.*

The chaplain is someone to hope with them. The bereaved need to know that the intense feeling of pain will subside and that they can withstand the pressure of waiting. They need reassurance that with time and effort the pain will go away.

I feel they need someone to hope for them because all too often their own sense of future dies with their loved one. Again, others who have experienced a similar loss, and who have progressed through the early phases of grief, and who have caught a glimpse of light at the end of the tunnel, can be the best sources of hope.

Rebuilding *can* take place. The bereaved need *someone to believe in them*, someone to say that it *is* worth the effort, that *they* are worth the effort. The pain of grief is such and the task of rebuilding is so overwhelming that there can be extreme self-doubt. Bereaved people can be very ambivalent as to whether their own lives are worth saving. Family members or friends may themselves begin to question whether the bereaved will ever get over their grief. In order to hasten recovery, they frequently put pressure on the bereaved by making unnecessary and unrealistic demands, such as not to show any emotion, not to talk about the deceased, not to visit the cemetery, and the like. Someone who believes in them can help the bereaved move through (without pushing them through) their grief.

There needs to be *someone to be honest with them*, someone to provide firm and consistent reminders that the loved one *is* dead and will never come back. It is important to do this within the context of remembering. Grievers will frequently confuse acceptance with forgetting. Accepting is not forgetting (and they may be reassured that they will not forget), but it is being able to remember without the piercing pain. Reality can be underscored only as people are given opportunity to discuss and share the remotest as well as the most significant memory of the deceased. Such honesty requires someone who will encourage the bereaved to engage in any activity which reminds them of their life together with the deceased.

Conclusion

Most clergy have had considerable experience in ministering to the dying. Through Clinical Pastoral Education more clergy are now engaging in such a ministry under close supervision. They are being asked to reflect upon death, their own and others'. Experience in ministering to the dying without such disciplined reflection may allow defenses against the reality of death to develop that may later render that ministry inadequate and superficial.

We have learned that unless pastors are at peace with their own mortality, and its vast implications, they are not free to accompany others in their dying.

The hospital chaplain witnesses to certain truths about life and death. But many times personal beliefs are confused with more general truths (those which all must accept). The universal truths to which chaplains bear witness are obviously that everyone dies and that life does go on. These general truths, however, must be distinguished from specific articles of faith. Failure to make this distinction can lead to lack of respect for individual beliefs. It can also lead to subtle (or overt) manipulation of others to believe as I (we) believe rather than to help such persons clarify and solidify their own beliefs.

Chaplains are not responsible for other people's beliefs. They are responsible only for their own. As persons of faith, chaplains are often called to be witnesses to that personal faith. But a chaplain's personal faith is only a foundation through which others are helped to summon their own faith, to make choices about their own beliefs, about their own dying or grieving. Though we all feel helpless in the face of death, or at the mercy of circumstances beyond our control, there are nevertheless choices to be made. In such ministry, the chaplain's task is to help others to find those areas where individual choices can be made while, at the same time, helping them to accept those larger, universal truths over which they have no control.

NOTES

1. Elisabeth Kübler-Ross, *On Death and Dying* (New York: MacMillan, 1969).

2. Avery D. Weisman, *On Dying and Denying* (New York: Behavioral Publications, Inc., 1972).

3. Ronald Ramsey, *Living With Loss* (New York: Morrow, 1981).

4. John Bowlby, *Attachment and Loss* (New York: Basic Books, 1969).

13

The Voices on Psychiatry: Inner Tumult and the Quest for Meaning

WILLARD WAGNER

"Pastor, can I talk to you?"

"Pastor, do you have some time, I have something that I need to discuss?"

"So you're the minister! I didn't think that I'd ever see someone like you in a place like this. I've got to see you."

It often begins that way on a psychiatric unit. Some approach me hesitantly. Others in desperation. Most are afraid — frightened both by the tumult of their inner world, as well as by the confusion and strangeness of their new outer world, a psychiatric unit. Some of the requests come with a sense of urgency, as if their return to health depended on this singular visit. At times the requests come with an undertone of anger. What the pastor symbolizes to them becomes a lightning rod that attracts emotional charges. It doesn't matter that this is our first meeting; the residual images are enough. At other times the tone is one of suspicion. Past betrayals, real or imagined, impede the present encounter. Some come willingly, expectant and hopeful; others come grudgingly, on orders of the psychiatrist.

These requests for pastoral care come in many different ways. Some are spoken loudly and directly. Others come indirectly, from other patients. Most often the requests come when chaplains make themselves physically and emotionally available.

Why Patients Seek Out a Chaplain

One reason that emotionally ill persons are able to make such requests is that many come out of a *community of faith*. In a weekly Faith and Life discussion group that a chaplain conducts on the psychiatric unit of Lutheran General Hospital, patients share their faith background and their current relationship to that faith. The stories will vary. For some, contact with a faith community has been extensive: "I went to a Catholic grade school and high school, and I remember as a small child going to church with my parents. Going to church on Sunday was as much a part of our life as eating meals and going to work." For others it was casual: "I grew up in a Jewish home. We didn't go to temple every week, but we would go on the high holy days and I went to Hebrew school. I had to do that before I could be Bar Mitzvahed. I don't go much anymore now that I've moved away from home. Once in a while I think about going to temple on Friday evening but mostly I go on one of the holy days." And for others it was only a brief encounter: "My mother used to send me to Sunday school, but that stopped when she got a divorce. The pastor from the church came to visit her, but after that I didn't go anymore."

The memories of those encounters and relationships impel them now to turn to a chaplain (a symbol of their pastor, priest, or rabbi) in time of trouble. From that community of faith many have experienced caring and nurturing, which they now hope to experience again from the chaplain. The chaplain on a psychiatric unit builds upon those early religious foundations. For the majority of the patients, that faith community and its leaders have included people they could trust and confide in.

For others those relationships have been negative, characterized by the patients as distrustful and uncaring. Such patients are more than willing to tell their "war stories" about past hurts. Yet surprisingly, they are still willing to confide in the chaplain. Is it an attempt to strike back, to wrest some revenge through the chaplain? Or is it a test, to see if the chaplain will respond like past religious authorities, by abandoning them? So they come with anger and hope. They wonder whether this chaplain will be there for them.

A second reason such people seek out a pastor is *a desperate need to be heard.* They feel afraid and overwhelmed. Often, too, they feel guilty. Many are suicidal. Some of them have shared their suicidal thoughts with others; some have attempted suicide and have been rushed to the hospital by the police or paramedics.

As a result of that thought or act, the patient is often filled with guilt. The presence of the chaplain at times both stimulates the guilt and gives them the opportunity to voice it. Though rarely spoken aloud, such people crave to hear words of understanding, acceptance, and comfort. At these moments, patients find it terribly hard to accept themselves, and the chaplain provides that moment of acceptance and acceptability. Sometimes it comes by a word, sometimes in a deed. Most often it comes by being with them and listening as they share their pain. The targets for their intense anger are many: family, friends, employers and fellow employees, God, but mostly themselves.

A third reason patients seek out a chaplain is *in response to the chaplain's initiative*. At Lutheran General Hospital the chaplain attempts to visit all psychiatric patients (see chap. 6 above). In this initial contact the chaplain and the chaplain's role on the unit are identified. In response to such initiative patients will seek out the chaplain with personal concerns.

A fourth reason that patients at times ask to speak with the chaplain comes from *the chaplain's involvement in the program activities* that take place on the psychiatric unit. Chaplains often serve as co-leaders in group therapy and attend team and community meetings. As a part of the multidisciplinary treatment team, patients come to know and experience the pastor from a new perspective. Their most common concept is that "pastors" serve a local congregation. So it is at times with surprise that they come to know the pastor as one who is in their midst, who has therapeutic understanding and concern. As a result of seeing the chaplain in a variety of unit functions, they seek out the chaplain with a variety of needs.

However, regardless of how or why the encounter occurs — whether out of memories of a faith community, a need to be heard, or in response to the chaplain's initiative or as a part of the treatment team — it is crucial that the chaplain be a sensitive, trusting, caring, responsive listener.

The Chaplain in a Supportive Ministry

A primary task in ministry to the emotionally ill is to discern the needs of the patient. It is vital that the chaplain's ministry be to those discerned needs, not out of any patented style of ministry the chaplain finds comfortable. In visiting the emotionally ill person the chaplain needs to ask: What is the patient saying to me? What is the patient needing from me at this moment? Can I provide what is needed for this patient? If I am unable to provide what is needed how can I mobilize other resources of help?

There are those times when the best that one can provide is a "supportive" ministry. By "supportive" is meant a specific counseling approach

which employs methods that seek to stabilize, undergird, nurture, moti-
vate, or guide troubled persons, enabling them to handle their problems and relationships more constructively within whatever limits are
imposed by their personality resources and circumstances.[1]

The goal in supportive ministry is to help persons cope with their present situation by more effectively utilizing their inner strengths as well as
the outer resources that are available to them. The focus of this ministry
is on the here and now; a major therapeutic resource is the variety of
relationships available on the unit and in the patient's intimate social
network. To help to restore and strengthen those relationships is a vital
goal of supportive ministry.

In supportive counseling we "lend" our ego, our strength, our wisdom
to troubled persons in order to help them to better utilize their own resources and to regain a sense of equilibrium.[2] Psychiatrist Franz Alexander describes five procedures that are used in supportive ministry:

1. *Emotional Catharsis.* Allowing the troubled person to pour out
one's feelings to another who listens and seeks to understand. Not only
does this provide emotional relief but it allows that person to overcome
loneliness by sharing the burden.

2. *Gratify Dependency Needs.* The pastor becomes a "good parent,"
upon whom the person can lean. As any "good parent" the counselor
will guide, instruct, and set proper limits and in so doing the patient will
be temporarily relieved of the full responsibility for responding to life.

3. *Aid the Ego Defenses.* Instead of probing or confronting, instead
of challenging defenses, the counselor will support those defenses which
are enabling the person to hold together during the crisis.

4. *Objective View of the Stress Situation.* An important aspect of
supportive ministry is to provide an objective overview of the immediate
crisis. This enables the person to more realistically explore alternative
options and to make appropriate decisions.

5. *Modifying the Life Situation.* On occasion it becomes necessary to
change the environment or to remove one from the environment so that the
person has a better chance to recover personal strengths and resources. In a
sense, a psychiatric hospitalization is an environmental manipulation
intended to temporarily remove one from the stresses and burdens of
one's life.[3]

In an age that hallows insight and in-depth psychotherapy, many
view supportive or sustaining counseling as superficial. But a supportive

ministry requires a great deal of sensitivity and compassion, both of the patient and of oneself. In offering a supportive ministry one has to contend not only with the patient's pain but with one's own anxiety as well. There is always the anxiety to do or to say something, to take away the patient's pain. Supportive ministry is often patient, quiet listening, allowing the patient's own resources and strength to emerge.

One of the key elements in a supportive ministry is compassion. Compassion is derived from the Latin *cum* ("with") and *passio* ("suffering"). Compassion means "suffering with."

In *If God Is Love—A Christian's Journey Through Suffering* Edna Hong writes: "Compassion means placing my 'I' in the sad or miserable or aching body of a fellow-being. A compassionate person is one who says, 'I am a part of this whole suffering world.' "[4]

There are several emotional illnesses where the very best and most meaningful ministry that the chaplain can provide is a supportive ministry—"a suffering with."

One of these is depression where the treatment of choice is either medication or electroshock therapy. Patients suffering from intense depression have little ability to concentrate on anything other than the pain they are experiencing. Generally, this type of depression is seen as a biological condition requiring medical intervention. Though there are also important psychosocial aspects, psychotherapy is often ineffective until the severe depression is relieved.

Recently, a patient came on the unit who was severely depressed for no apparent reason. There had been no recent loss or disappointment. It was learned, however, that a number of relatives in his family had also suffered from severe depressive episodes. It was decided that medication, or drug therapy, would be the treatment of choice. In the meantime, this patient was still left with the inward pain created by the depression. He knew that he was not functioning at work or relating to his family. The despair was overpowering. "I feel like I'm standing on the edge of a dark, bottomless pit and at any time now I'm likely to fall into the pit and I have no control over when that will happen." These moments of despair were terrifying to the patient. Though he was receiving the prescribed medication, it had not as yet had time to take full effect. My role as pastor was to be with the patient, to listen as he poured out his pain and doubts. "Do you think this medication will do any good?" "How long will I have to suffer this way?" "I don't see any purpose in this; I know that God cares for me; I know his love. That's the one thing that I continue to hang onto, but how long?"

Listening and giving encouragement ("Yes, indeed, the medication will help; God's love and care of us is present even in the midst of despair; yes, there will come moments of calm and relief from the overwhelming despair.") were my primary ministry. In due time the medication did take effect; the grip of the depression did let go, and he was able to return home and shortly thereafter to return to work.

One brief incident that he reported later, after hospitalization, supports the concept that what he needed from the chaplain was a supportive ministry. He reported that during his hospitalization he was assigned a student nurse who was to relate to him on a one-to-one basis. Initially, she spent time with him and listened to him as he poured out his words and tears. He appreciated her willingness to be with him. Later in his stay, she began to do some library research to learn more about his kind of depression and the medication he was taking. Now armed with this new-found knowledge, she returned to spend time with him, only now she had answers to give, hoping that these answers would be helpful. But it had just the opposite effect. The patient reported that from then on he felt less close to her. Where before he was delighted to see her and spend time with her, now he wanted her to leave him alone.

A second group which can benefit from a supportive ministry consists of those who have religious delusions. When a patient announces to me that she is the bride of Christ, or another that he is a prophet sent by God to warn us of the end of the world, then I take that as my cue to be as supportive as I can. The hard work for the chaplain is *to support the person but not the delusion.*

Recently a patient requested to see me and insisted that we go into an office where we would be alone: "Pastor, I know that I haven't done what God wanted me to do, but do you think that he will give me back my brain ? I feel that this is God's punishment for what I did wrong; he came down and plucked my brain right out of my head. Do you think he'll give it back to me?"

This patient fervently believed that this act of God is what caused him to be admitted to a psychiatric unit. When God gave him back his brain, then he would be allowed to return home. My pastoral stance was to focus not on the delusion and any possible dynamic interpretations, but rather to support the reality of God's continued love and care for him.

A third group of patients for whom a supportive ministry is most appropriate are those patients who are admitted to the psychiatric unit with an organic mental disorder that has caused major changes in both behavior and personality. As a result of these changes the patient is admitted to the hospital by the family in order to determine the cause for this unusual behavior.

There are a number of different diseases that cause organic changes in the brain, such as multiple strokes, Alzheimer's disease, and Pick's disease. Presently, there is little that can be done to change the degenerative progression of these diseases and thus the appropriate pastoral stance is to support the patient and the family. Both need support as they begin to face the consequences of a disorder that slowly and insidiously causes multifaceted losses of memory, reasoning, and changes in personality and behavior. They also need support as they proceed to make decisions about treatment and their future together. The chaplain can play a supportive role by identifying community resources available to them, such as home care, or respite care.

The Chaplain in a Dialogic Ministry

There are those persons who not only need to be supported in their times of emotional crisis but also they need help to explore their inner world in order to make sense out of what seems to be nonsense, to find meaning in the midst of what appears initially to be a meaningless experience. Such a quest is best met through a ministry of dialogue, in which the chaplain and the patient engage in a mutual exploration of the dynamic meaning behind the patient's bizarre feelings and behavior.

In the dialogic ministry trust is often initially invested in the chaplain's symbolic role. As the relationship develops, trust and confidence are experienced at an interpersonal level. It is at this point that the chaplain attempts to blend a symbolic pastoral role with a pastoral counseling role. That is, the chaplain begins with whatever his or her presence stimulates in terms of images and memories from past experiences with clergy and/or other authorities, and gradually enables the patient to transfer that confidence, to respond to current reality-based relationships, such as the one being established between the patient and the chaplain.

Mrs. L. was a sixty-two-year-old patient who was seen shortly after being admitted to the locked psychiatric unit. I had barely finished introducing myself when she blurted out: "Oh pastor, everything has gone wrong and it's all my fault. It's all because I told a lie and now everyone will find out and I'll be ruined, my husband will be ruined and we'll lose everything."

This relationship began on a confessional level. The patient's past experiences with clergy indicated to her that the confession of guilt was an appropriate way to initiate a relationship with a pastor.

When I asked her if she could share with me what happened, she quickly did. When she was six years old, her father had committed suicide. As the years passed, whenever she was asked about her father's death, she was too ashamed to tell the truth, so she told everyone that he had died of TB. The only person with whom she had shared the truth about her father's death was her husband. About a month prior to her admission to the hospital, her son-in-law had been killed in a car accident. In her guilt she immediately concluded that his tragic death resulted from her "great lie." One of the phrases that she repeated was, "Now my husband will lose everything—I'll be put away and he'll lose everything in order to pay the bills."

In our initial sessions together she continued to focus on her "lie" and how this hospitalization was God's punishment for it. Later, in a meeting with the patient, her husband, and the social worker, it became clear that she was upset and angry not only about the deaths of her father and son-in-law but also with her recently retired husband who was now around the house all day. This disturbed her, but being a "good Christian" she could not bring herself to express such feelings to him. She felt the need for some separation from him, but was fearful that expressing her anger would hurt him. We began to pursue her relationship with her husband, her deep ambivalence about his retirement, her need for space, and her fears of losing him if she claimed such space and expressed her real feelings.

We discussed the bind this put her in and how she was turning the anger in on herself. We also discussed her lack of trust in her husband's capacity to tolerate such feelings and of the lack of trust she had in the durability of the relationship. We talked about the power of love and the freedom of truth. Gradually, she came to trust her relationships with me and with others on the unit. She found that she could be both open and acceptable. In due time she was able to be open to her own and her husband's feelings. She became more expressive and had less need to punish herself. Her depression lifted and she went home.

This ministry began with a confession. But rather than take the confession totally at face value, an attempt was made to get at other feelings that were tied in with her "sin." The guilt over concealing her father's suicide was heard and accepted, but she also was helped to see that her current feelings toward her husband were stronger contributors to her depression than her guilt for a childhood incident. Indeed, her ambivalence over intimacy issues and her fears of losing her husband as she once lost her father were explored and interpreted.

This ministry of dialogue takes place not only between patient and pastor but also, as it did for Mrs. L., with other staff and patients and family. In fact, the chaplain-patient relationship is but a microcosm of other relationships that are or need to be developing. In our psychiatric unit peer group sharing is a daily and highly valued activity.

Dialogue also took place between pastor and treatment team in order to effectively coordinate the treatment goals for Mrs. L. It is through ongoing dialogue that trust is built among members of the interdisciplinary treatment team.

The Chaplain as Teacher

When people come to that point in their lives when they need to be admitted to a psychiatric facility, they begin to raise serious questions about their relationship to God. In the midst of such crises people of faith are searching for new meanings to some age-old questions. In this search, some attempt to "put new wine into old wine skins," while others search for a belief system that will hold this painful event in their lives without bursting the seams.

The chaplain is given a multitude of opportunities to teach. Sometimes it takes place in the weekly Faith and Life discussion group where patients have an opportunity to share their faith concerns with one another; at other times, when patients seek out the chaplain as "the religious expert."

Recently, a psychiatrist referred a patient to the chaplain who saw God as a source of punishment. The physician's request: "Can you help Joe to understand that God is different than the way he presently views him?" Joe was willing to share his story, for this was the third time that he had been hospitalized for recurring depression. But this time, Joe's story included parts he had not shared in his previous hospitalizations:

> Pastor, I know that I belong here because God punishes those who have sinned. That's what I was taught as I grew up. I went to a Catholic grade school and that was the message I learned from the nuns: "If you sin God will punish you," and I feel that I have really sinned. It happened fifteen years ago when I was dating the woman who became my wife. We had sexual relations and she became pregnant and then I forced her to get an abortion. Now, pastor, I don't know the Bible as well as I should, but I do know that what I did was wrong. I took a life. I feel I deserve what I've been getting because of what I did.

During the four weeks that Joe remained in the hospital the chaplain met with him three to four times a week to talk about the God against whom he had sinned. In the initial sessions Joe spent much time sharing his sorrow for his behavior. But then attention shifted to God whom Joe perceived to be angry. The chaplain began to cite biblical passages which spoke of God's enduring mercy. Joe would counter with biblical references of God's condemnation. For instance, one day the chaplain shared John 3:16: "God so loved the world. . . ." The next day Joe announced that he had read the entire third chapter of John and from it quoted: "our deeds are evil and therefore we deserve punishment."

Joe's countering pointed to a need for reassurance. Slowly he came to see that judgment and mercy were both attributes of God. Slowly he came to see these in balance. As God's love was brought to the surface, Joe began to see that he was an object of such love. Joe received that message in several ways: through the verbal teaching of God's truth, through hearing the message and beginning to integrate it into his life, and also through the consistency of the chaplain's presence. In some ways, the pastor became an embodiment of those words, making them concrete, believable, and attainable. It was as if Joe was saying, "If I am so terrible, then why is this person caring for me?" Thus the message was taught and caught through a personal presence.

However, that message was also conveyed through the presence of the Holy Spirit who was there, as Paul promised he would be in his letter to the Romans (8:16-17): "It is the Spirit Himself bearing witness with our spirit that we are children of God, and if children, then heirs, heirs of God and fellow heirs with Christ, provided we suffer with Him in order that we also be glorified with Him."

Sometimes the opportunity to teach comes when patients question their faith because of inability to conquer their emotional problems. "Pastor, I can't understand how I ended up here. I have a strong faith in God and I was always taught that if I truly believe then everything would be all right in my life. Maybe my faith wasn't as strong as I thought it was." When such issues are raised, the chaplain again has the opportunity to teach through both words and personal presence. It is only when word and presence come together—when these two dimensions are congruent—that the patient can begin to come to a new understanding of one's faith. Such moments can be occasions to help people understand and accept their human nature, their imperfections, their vulnerabilities, their mistakes, and doubts. Many people of faith tend to see emotional illness as something a strong faith should have repelled. Many such people are gratified to hear that invincibility, mental health, emotional stability are not always accompaniments of faith. It is also reassuring for such people to be reminded that God's acceptance of them is total, including their immaturities and instabilities.

A patient often says that "the church taught me." Sometimes patients state this with a sense of joy and the teachings are a source of strength. If these teachings seem realistic and appropriate for the patient's current situation, the chaplain reinforces such teachings. At other times, patients relate their understanding of the church's teaching with irritation or confusion. The chaplain allows such feelings to be expressed, without attempting to defend the church or to reprimand the expressions. More often than not when such negative expressions go unchallenged, the patients are then freed to express the positive side of their ambivalent feelings toward the church. Many such people are trapped in their relationship to the church. They have many memories of its perceived failing and, at times, harsh teachings, but their deep loyalty will not allow them to sever their relationship to it. A chaplain can help such ambivalence to be expressed. As patients are helped to see and to accept their human failings and strengths, so they are often helped to see that the church is both divine and human.

The Church's Challenge

The church and its pastors are provided some rich opportunities for ministry in periods of emotional illness. In 1920, Anton Boisen, one of the first full-time mental hospital chaplains and the father of Clinical Pastoral Education, wrote, "In many of its forms, insanity as I see it, is a religious rather than a medical problem, and any treatment which fails to recognize that fact can hardly be effective. But as yet the Church has given little attention to this problem."[5] In the years that have passed since Anton Boisen wrote those words the church has given considerable attention to the problem of "insanity" in all of its forms, and yet a great deal remains to be done. There is still much fear and misunderstanding on the part of people when they are faced with one who is seriously ill emotionally. People continue to have distorted concepts about the causes and cures of emotional problems. Anton Boisen had a part of the truth when he made his assessment over sixty years ago that emotional illness is a religious problem, but I think he was only partially correct. Emotional illness is not only a religious problem, it's a medical, social, and psychological one as well. We who represent the church as chaplains need to take an active role in proclaiming that truth to those who suffer from emotional illnesses and to those who are a part of the communities of faith from which such people come.

NOTES

1. Howard J. Clinebell, *Basic Types of Pastoral Counseling* (Nashville: Abington Press, 1966), p. 139.

2. Ibid., p. 141.

3. Franz Alexander, *Psychoanalysis and Psychotherapy* (New York: W. W. Norton, Inc., 1956), pp. 55-56.

4. Edna Hong, *If God Is Love—A Christian's Journey through Suffering* (Minneapolis: Augsburg Publishing House, 1978), p.44.

5. R. C. Powell, *Anton T. Boisen, Breaking an Opening in the Wall between Religion and Medicine* (New York: Association of Mental Health Clergy, 1976), p.8.

14

The Voices of Substance Abuse:
A Spiritual Perspective

CARL ANDERSON

Compulsive destructive drinking patterns have puzzled observers of the human condition for centuries. Persons who did not themselves experience a powerful craving for alcohol typically viewed "drunkards" as weak-willed, irresponsible people, intentionally "drowning their sorrows." The gradual acceptance of mental disorders as legitimate illnesses in the twentieth century resulted in the view that "chronic inebriates" were suffering from an underlying mental disorder. Many people in the various health professions, including many of the clergy, were trained to view excessive drinking, or other mood-altering substance dependence, as a symptom of some underlying personality problem. Even this ostensibly enlightened view did not offer much hope to the chemically dependent person as therapists failed dismally in attempting to help with this approach.

Although there have been other attempts to treat alcohol dependence as a disease, the movement which has had the most significant impact is Alcoholics Anonymous, which traces its beginnings to the spiritual awakening and subsequent recovery of "Dr. Bob" and Bill W.[1]

While AA and its many derivative groups have had unparalleled success in treating addictive disorders, the debate continues, both among professionals and lay people, as to whether alcoholism, or any of the drug dependencies, are legitimate diseases.[2] While there is increasing evidence of genetic biochemical factors, it is widely accepted that social, cultural, psychological, and spiritual factors are also present.[3]

How can clergy and other professionals best understand this strange affliction? I would suggest that addictive illnesses are best understood from a *spiritual perspective* that includes both genetic and environmental factors. This view accepts the fact that some individuals are predisposed due to genetic variables and therefore more vulnerable to certain addictions. It also posits that all human beings are prone to addictive disorders. According to this perspective, susceptibility to addictive illness is rooted in our spiritual condition.

The view of human nature described in Genesis is that people are created for relationship. This design makes us dependent upon God and other people if we are to experience full humanity. The core of sin (the fall) is rebellion against, or the rejection of, our state of dependence. Instead, security is sought in power and control, rather than in dependence upon and trust in intangible faith relationships. *The anxiety and insecurity that results from our attempts to live apart from faith relationships is the soil out of which addiction grows.* This attempt to live apart from faith relationships is a universal phenomenon; all human beings experience the feeling of being anxious and fearful of being alone and limited. Our human dilemma is that we are created for relationship; our most basic human needs can only be met through relationships with others, yet we strive to find some other way.

Any substance or activity that promises the possibility of the reduction of those feelings is highly attractive, especially if the experience is one that is fairly tangible and appears controllable. There is an almost overwhelming urge in human beings to find some way of feeling secure, happy, and in control of their destiny. As we grow and develop, most of us encounter at least one thing or activity that makes us feel the way we want to feel, at least temporarily. Food, sex, power, money, alcohol or other drugs are common attractions. The existence of harmful dependencies and/or addictions to these substances or activities are very real in human life.

These dependencies are best understood as rooted in the human spiritual dilemma. In our quest for more apparent freedom, in our desire to feel good, we turn to things that ultimately decrease freedom and diminish human fullness. Repeated use of one or more of these "feel good" activities, or substances, can easily progress to a psychological dependence, and depending on individual differences, to a compulsive harmful addiction. At this addictive level the individual loses the ability to reverse or control the pattern by choice. The activity or substance that once was an ally and friend has become a powerful master that dominates choice and assumes priority over human relationships. Addition to alcohol, or other mood-altering substances, is more frequent and visible than other addictions due to the profound effect of the drug(s) on the central nervous system.

Most people who abuse alcohol over a long enough period of time will develop an addiction to it. Sudden withdrawal of the drug will result in physical disturbance as well as emotional panic. For some people, alcohol (or another drug) provides a "magic" or special "high" from the first experience that is markedly different from that of others. In some cases, these people may appear to be in control of the experience for some years. In reality, they are "hooked" almost immediately and will progress into more obvious addictive symptoms if they continue to engage in the activity.

There has been much argument over the years, which continues to the present time, over whether the development of addiction is due primarily to psychological or physical factors. While researchers differ on this question, there is a growing consensus that many alcoholics have a genetic predisposition to their condition. Yet, in all probability, alcoholism and other drug dependencies are not due to one single cause. Depending on one's point of view, many causes may be identified. For example, there seems to be little debate over the fact that most alcoholics experience a very positive reaction to alcohol or some other drug. Without this positive reaction, it is almost impossible to develop an addiction to it. There is almost universal agreement among researchers that offspring of alcoholics do experience a higher rate of addiction to alcohol or other drugs than offspring of nonalcoholic parents. Some, however, argue that this can be explained by social and environmental factors as well as genetic. In my opinion, the best understanding of alcoholism and drug addiction comes through the acceptance of multiple causality, which allows for genetic, psychological, social, and spiritual factors.

Addiction: A Disease or a Symptom?

Is this addictive pattern a disease, or is it a symptom of another disorder? Might addiction be a convenient excuse for irresponsible behavior? Certainly addictive illnesses are not infectious diseases like pneumonia or influenza. But in the broader concept of illness, which includes conditions in which the individual is unable to function normally and cannot decide to be well (similar to colds, hay fever, or heart disease), the alcoholic or drug-dependent person is indeed sick. As in many illnesses, hindsight may clearly identify contributing factors, *but knowledge of these does not change the present reality of the condition once it has developed.*

What about the common view that alcoholism is a symptom of a deeper psychological disorder which also needs treatment? Sometimes it is; usually it is not. Due to the behavioral nature of this illness, the alcoholic is frequently observed to be depressed, grandiose, impatient, impulsive or moody. For most alcoholics, these symptoms are part of the illness and respond naturally to the spiritual therapy that is experienced in the fellowship of AA and by using the twelve steps of AA in daily living. There are, however, persons for whom additional therapy is needed for underlying or concurrent psychological or living problems.

Is the disease concept an excuse? Hardly! No individual or family member affected by this illness enjoys it. Most are desperate for help. Clergy who grasp the spiritual nature and effects of this illness are often in an excellent position to offer that help. One important need is for clergy and other professionals to be knowledgeable about the typical symptoms of an alcohol or drug problem.

Warning Signs of Alcohol/Drug Dependence

Alcohol and/or other drug dependence may be defined as *a harmful dependence on any mood-altering substance.* This dependence is characterized by repeated use despite negative consequences; a progression in the amount, frequency of use, and harmful effects; and an inability to moderate use of the substance according to healthy patterns. The following are warning signs of progressive alcohol/drug dependence:

1. *Preoccupation*	looking forward to the pleasurable effect (like being in love)
2. *Rapid Use*	quick ingestion to obtain the chemical effect, sneaking drinks while making drinks for others, drinking doubles, drinking before a party, etc.
3. *Hiding*	the dependent person panics at the thought of being without, so a supply is kept safely concealed

4. *Solitary Use*	solitary drinking or drinking with groups in bars while "alone" emotionally
5. *Tolerance*	developing a greater capacity (three to four drinks needed for the same effect one or two used to have)
6. *Unpredictability*	the amount or effect is greater than intended
7. *Memory Blackout*	periods of time in which the user may function normally but cannot remember what was said or done
8. *Universality*	most any occasion is a good time to drink or use (i.e., happy times to celebrate, tense times to relax, sad times to forget, etc.)

The specific symptoms will vary according to the person's age and life pattern. For most people, work or school life will be the most carefully protected. If problems appear at school or work, the illness is usually present. Some people may develop physical problems (liver disease, gastritis, pancreatitis, etc.) relatively early in their progression; others, later. This variability is true in all problem areas: family, social, and emotional. The primary clue to watch for is a pattern of negative change in the person's functioning that is associated with alcohol or drug use.

Intervention

Most helping professionals have experienced the frustration of clearly identifying an alcohol or drug problem and not knowing for sure how to intervene effectively. Frequently, the person with the identified problem is highly resistant to suggestions for help. Often the family members are distraught and upset about the problem, but are also very frightened by the alcoholic's threats and negative responses when the problem is raised by them. The most common request made to a chaplain, parish pastor, or other professional is: "Help us to do something about the person's drinking, but don't rock the boat."

Chaplains in hospital settings frequently feel great frustration in assisting patients or family members with a substance abuse problem. The emotional accessibility of the patient or family member is limited. This can be due to denial, guilt, or fear of rocking the boat or provoking a disturbance. Other professionals frequently have a limited knowledge of substance abuse problems and do not support a treatment plan that includes addressing possible substance abuse. Chaplains do have a unique opportunity to minister effectively in these situations, since patients, family members, and staff expect the chaplain to be involved in personal problems. This expectation does provide an opportunity to address problems of substance abuse.

The most important beginning step in any intervention is to recognize that the family profoundly suffers from this illness in ways that make it difficult for them to respond effectively. For this reason, it is important not to jump too quickly into an intervention process before the family is ready. One of the best referrals any helping professional can make for a family is to Al-Anon. Family members may need considerable encouragement and support to begin this involvement because they typically fear the alcoholic's response. Other family members will report that they went to a few meetings and it did not seem to help. The chaplain at this point must understand that the family is trapped by feelings of fear and hopelessness, and by their perceptions that the urgent need is to fix or change the alcoholic/substance abuser. Patient guidance, explanations, and reading material can be sources of support to the family. [4]

Chaplains themselves should go to open Al-Anons and AA meetings to gain understanding of the recovery process. All chaplains should know how to make an effective Al-Anon referral. It is often best to give the family members a phone number and offer them the opportunity to call for a referral from your office. It is also helpful to know some Al-Anon members in your community who are willing to share their experience with a newcomer and even to take them to a meeting. Families Anonymous is a similar fellowship for parents and siblings of young alcoholics or drug abusers. It is excellent support and guidance for families who are feeling angry, bewildered, guilty, frustrated, and hopeless.

It cannot be overstated that the most effective intervention in most situations of alcoholism or other drug dependence is *to help the family free itself from feeling trapped by the illness and to begin making positive changes in its own response to the illness*. Even though the alcoholic may threaten, plead, and cajole the family to do otherwise, the family that firmly resolves to begin new behavior patterns will experience personal freedom and create a much more realistic situation for the problem drinker. Once the problem drinker or drug user begins to realize that the family will no longer continue to shield or to remove the consequences from his or her unrealistic behavior, change is much more likely to occur.

Most communities have out-patient clinics and service agencies that offer structured intervention programs for alcoholics and drug abusers. Unless the chaplain or other helping professional wants to specialize in this kind of work, it is probably unwise to do more than to identify the problem and to make a referral. Professionals who specialize in this work can be much more effective in providing the much needed help.

Moral Considerations

Clergy specializing in alcoholism and drug abuse services are often asked what can be done to prevent the problem, rather than just treat it after it occurs. There is also the rather common view among many religious people that offering treatment for this illness implies acceptance of drug abuse in our society. Such critics will frequently point to the tremendous harm caused by alcohol and drug use in our society.

There is no question that modern society in most parts of the world has serious alcohol and drug abuse problems. The situations in North America, Europe, and Russia are especially well documented. Not only is there a serious health problem from the direct physical and psychological damage of abuse, the problems of drunk driving and lost time in the work place are increasingly severe. In the United States it is estimated that over one-half of all traffic fatalities are the direct consequence of alcohol and drug abuse. The leading cause of death among teenagers in our society is accidents, followed by suicide. It is estimated that 80 percent of these fatal accidents and 60 percent of the suicides are related to alcohol and drug abuse. Is it any surprise, then, that many responsible persons identify this as not only the number one health problem but also the number one *moral issue* in our society?

The question of effective prevention is extremely complex and elusive. One approach to prevention seeks to identify those individuals who are high risk for developing an alcohol/drug problem due to genetic factors and/or psychological/social problems. The difficulty with this approach is that no one knows for certain how to identify these factors;

and even if they were clearly known, how to persuade people to modify their behavior based on this knowledge. Another approach to prevention emphasizes alternative "highs" through physical exercise and social life, and stresses "responsible drinking" as a way of preventing future alcohol problems.

A third preventative approach is to encourage abstinence. This is seen by many as the best moral choice, given the high-risk rate for those who use alcohol or drugs and the apparent difficulty of preventing the development of problems among those who do.

Other people point out that for those who drink, only a small percentage develop problems with alcohol. They argue that, rather than encouraging abstinence, society should concentrate on identifying the etiological factors for that small percentage who have a problem with the moderate use of alcohol. Such people further argue that previous attempts to enforce wide-scale abstinence have failed.

There is evidence that families that have very moralistic feelings about alcohol use, and who practice total abstinence for moral reasons, have a high rate of problem drinking when family members choose to use alcohol at some point in their lives.

While there is no easy answer to this problem, the most rational approach is to examine the evidence as objectively as possible and take into account the various known factors. Since we know that some people are predisposed to the development of alcohol and/or drug problems, a society interested in the prevention of these problems would deglamorize the use of alcohol and/or drugs and teach young people a very cautious, moderate approach to their use. Moderate use would include religious and ceremonial use, low-percentage beverage alcohol as part of meals, careful use of alcohol at social functions, no impairing intoxication at any time, and all avoidance of alcohol/drug use to "prove" something or to cope with problems. Abstinence would be presented as a rational choice for those who wish to avoid problems. Those who choose to use alcohol or other drugs would make that choice in the light of factual knowledge about the effects of the drugs on the human body.

A society that has a nonmoralistic approach to the use/abstinence issue and that teaches and reinforces moderation as the expected norm for those who do choose its use will have an effective approach to prevention. If this approach will not totally eliminate alcohol and drug addiction, early and effective intervention is the best response to these problems once they have developed.

NOTES

1. Ernest Kurtz, *Not God* (Minneapolis: Hazelden Press, 1979). Kurtz gives a thorough analysis of the historical development of AA, identifying the spiritual foundations of this fellowship.

2. George E. Vaillant, *The Natural History of Alcoholism* (Cambridge: Harvard University Press, 1983), pp. 3–4. Chap. 1 discusses this issue at length.

3. Ibid., chap. 2.

4. John E. Keller, *Drinking Problem?* (Philadelphia: Fortress Press, 1971). This book is an excellent tool to use for self-diagnosis. Due to its clarity and brevity, it can be given to a problem drinker or family member for help in deciding whether or not a problem is present.

·PART III·

THE HOSPITAL CHAPLAIN:
Many Other Functions

15

The Chaplain as Administrator

LAWRENCE E. HOLST

"I don't want your chaplains discussing diagnosis with my patients before I do," intoned an irate physician.

"All budgets need to be cut by 5 percent in the next fiscal year," implored the vice-president for finances.

"The J.C.H.A. (Joint Commission on Hospital Accreditation) will be here next month; we'd better clarify our procedures on chaplains' use of patient charts," cautioned the director of medical records.

"Does our hospital have an ethical statement on the cessation of treatment?" inquired an oncology staff nurse.

"All division chiefs must complete their MBOs (management by objectives) by 30 June," stated the administrative memo.

"Maybe I'm just burned out," lamented the coronary care chaplain.

"Chaplain Burrow's six-month evaluation is past due," advised the director of personnel.

"With surgery's expansion, we're going to have to reassign some first floor offices," explained the management engineer.

"There's a lot of conflict among the staff chaplains about the weekend coverage schedule," warned the Division of Pastoral Care's secretary.

So the work goes for the pastoral administrator: trouble-shooting, budget managing, policy writing; formulating long-range plans, scheduling meetings, organizing agendas, resolving conflicts, evaluating work performances; listening, writing, processing, deciding. The purpose of it all is to provide and maintain the systems, structures, procedures, and organizations that will enable pastoral care to be delivered efficiently and effectively.

In most hospitals, the Division of Pastoral Care (or Chaplaincy Department) has a designated place in the institution's administrative hierarchy. Years ago, when chaplains and chaplaincy departments were fewer in number, little was expected of them administratively. Recent growth in size and numbers has resulted in expanded resources and services, which have necessitated more and better management, and its resultant increase in the administrative responsibilities of chaplains. If this means more inclusiveness in the hospital's organizational structure and more influence for pastoral care, it also means more conflict and competition with other department managers for budgets, space, and influence. To retain one's pastoral identity and demeanor in all of this is a challenge. Any hospital chaplain who fled the parish to escape administration is in for a rude awakening, even if the chaplain is spared the two major organizational tasks of the parish pastor: fund raising and new-member recruitment. The chaplain is part of an extremely complex bureaucracy, comprised of many well-trained professionals who provide an increasingly broad range of services. Unlike the parish, the primary focus of the hospital is not pastoral care. As well, it is an institution that is becoming increasingly overregulated and underfunded.

Parish and Hospital Administration Contrasted

Most hospital chaplains first experienced administration in the quite different context of the parish. In the parish it was much more difficult to separate the "clinical" delivery of pastoral care from administration. This was true because of the pastor's protracted proximity to the "consumer" (the parishioner). In the parish the consumer of pastoral services also directs those services. There is no real intermediary between deliverer and consumer. True, there are parish boards and committees, but these, too, are made up of consumers of pastoral services.

In hospital chaplaincy the relationship between the deliverer and receiver of services is more circumscribed. Their mutual accountability is confined to those "moments of ministry." That the chaplain and patient will have any other interactions outside that involvement is remote.

Not so in the parish. The breadth of mutual availability and mutual claims is quite unparalleled. The pastor has a multitude of roles and functions, most of which require the cooperation and support of the parishioner-consumer. The "spillage," or carry-over, from these interactions is inevitable. The parish pastor rarely has the luxury of ever being exclusively "a counselor," or "a teacher," or "a preacher," or "an administrator" to any parishioner. The pastor is all of these and more. Members of a parish, who are recipients of these pastoral services, serve on building committees, teach Sunday school, approve the pastor's salary and fringe benefits, allocate funds for parsonage improvements. All members cast important votes on issues that impact the life of that parish and its pastor. Many of these interactions may, and often do, place pastor and parishioner on opposite sides of issues.

At the same time, all of these members are recipients of pastoral care: they get sick, have weddings, baptisms and funerals, encounter marriage problems, get emotionally disturbed, have auto accidents, experience family conflicts. They will seek out and expect care from their pastor, whom they know well. Indeed, they may know their pastor so well from past administrative disagreements that it is difficult for them to receive ministry. The power and reprisals available on each side of the pastor-parishioner relationship—both direct and subtle, conscious and unconscious—are staggering. We avoid speaking of this. Perhaps we prefer not to face it or, in our naiveté, we assume that it will be easily subsumed under Christian love.

What further complicates matters is that the congregation's ministry is supported by voluntary contributions (not fees for services). Therefore, the parishioner-recipient exercises considerable control over those services and who provides them. Dissatisfaction with such services can be expressed in a variety of ways: by withholding contributions, by quitting the church, by mobilizing a dissent group. Since the parish is a fairly small, close community, such actions can quickly arouse attention. Such attention, in turn, can escalate conflicts that impede ministry and injure the pastor's standing in that community. These numerous and varied interactions between pastor and parishioner make it difficult to define and maintain neat administrative boundaries.

Pastoral administration in a hospital is quite different. For one thing, recipients of ministry (consumers of pastoral services) do not manage the hospital. That is, they don't occupy positions that empower them to evaluate or allocate funds for chaplaincy. True, board members and hospital administrators, who do manage the hospital, occasionally become patients in the hospital and receive pastoral care. But that is not the rule.

To be sure, hospital patients are not without a voice in such matters. They can, and do, complain and make suggestions. But they are not an organized, cohesive constituency. Nor are they voting members of hospital management. In addition, most hospital patients do not realize that they are paying for pastoral services. Certainly, that connection is not as obvious as the one between their Sunday offering and the parish pastor's salary.

A chaplain's administrative accountability is not to the patient. It is to an intermediary between the patient and the board, to a hospital administrator. The hospital's administrative network is the chaplain's constituency, the base line of support, not patients, however important they are. The chaplain's primary responsibility to the patient is to provide pastoral care. The relationships between them are confined to that basic delivery.

While the hospital context allows for "cleaner," more sharply defined pastor-patient relationships, it also deprives the chaplain of the visible support of those patients, who have known and experienced the chaplain's pastoral services. Seldom is there a movement in the community among former patients to establish, maintain, or expand hospital chaplaincy services.

An Important Implication

If the hospital chaplain's primary administrative responsibility is not to the patient but to a network of hospital administrators; and if this primary constituency does not usually experience or "consume" clinical pastoral services, then *this means that pastoral administration may provide that constituency with its only exposure to pastoral care.* The fact is that this network of hospital administrators' primary, first-hand experience with pastoral care is around administrative matters: meetings attended, plans formulated, disagreements resolved, commitments followed up, authority exercised.

If pastoral administration is a primary means for building constituency support, then it follows that chaplains ought to work at being good administrators. In a sense, the task of attaining administrative competency is not unlike that of the chaplain attaining clinical competency. Since the chaplain will interact with those who are trained and skilled in administration, the challenge will be to draw upon their knowledge and methods and to integrate that data around and within one's pastoral identity.

Are Pastoral Care and Administration Incompatible?

The word *administer* comes from the same root word as *ministry* (e.g., to administer the sacraments). May we not then infer that to administrate is to minister, to serve?

Clearly, there can be no ministry without administration. Even in a one-chaplain department time must be budgeted, needs discerned, resources allocated, effectiveness evaluated. No department, no community, no society can survive without some order and direction. Since administration is a universal human requirement, no one can speak of standing above or outside it. In ordination we speak of "setting apart," of being authorized to do things that are exclusive and unique. Administration points to functions that are common to all of us. For we are all administrators of something. Our survival depends on it.

To administer one must have authority. Authority tends to follow skills that meet recognized human needs.[1] A physician's authority is taken for granted. Physicians do not have to make a case for medicine's importance. Likewise, lawyers have recognized skills that confer authority. A hospital administrator rarely needs to make a case for administration. The growing complexity of health care delivery clearly speaks of that need.

What is the source of the pastor's authority? No doubt there was a time when the social framework gave natural and institutional reinforcement to the function and importance of ministry.[2] Unlike the physician, the lawyer, and the hospital administrator, the chaplain cannot count upon the exercise of skills as a valid source of authority. Many would not admit to a need for those skills. *The pastor's only claim to authority comes from representing God's claim over all of life.* To deny that claim, as many in society do, is to cut out the ground from pastoral authority. The chaplain's is *a representative authority*. It is not based upon a particular set of skills that a society, or a hospital, absolutely requires to fulfill its vital functions.

The danger that a chaplain-administrator may overclaim that representative authority is enormous. Certainly, such authority does not ensure infallibility in administrative decisions. Because the pastor's authority is seen as divinely representative, there is a strong expectation that a pastor's character, attitude, temperament, judgments, and behavior be consistent with that source of authority. To many, only such characteristics validate such authority. Granted, this is dangerous ground because it could lead to the presumption, unfair to them and to others, that pastors are morally superior. Yet, as representatives of God (upon which authority is claimed) it is a legitimate expectation that chaplains will bring to their administrative tasks the values and convictions inherent in their faith. Inconsistencies between profession and practice do raise doubts about the validity of that representative claim.

In one sense, a chaplain's administration is a means to an end: it is a means of making the clinical delivery of pastoral care in the hospital more effective and efficient. In another sense, a chaplain's administration is an end in itself: *it is pastoral care.* It is ministry, bringing something of the claims of God to the concrete world of things and people. Just as God's grace became more fully known through an earthly incarnation, so ministry becomes "incarnate" by touching mundane realities such as budgets, policies, procedures, requisitions, and memos. Either these all belong to God, or we must carefully define those areas that exclude him. How these duties are performed is an important aspect of ministry.

When one looks at a pastor's administrative functions, it becomes clearer that ministry is both a "calling" and a "profession." "Calling" defines the source, character, and goals of ministry; it is the basis for ministry. But one's "calling" to ministry ought never be a rationalization for professional incompetence. For ministry is also a "profession," requiring skills that must be learned and competencies that must be mastered, even if a pastor's "professionalism" ought never be a rationalization for lack of faith. Skills and competencies enable a pastor to translate a calling into a relevant, meaningful profession. Yet skills and competencies are only tools, not the substance and goals of ministry. Such substance and goals come from the source of one's calling, from the one upon whom pastoral authority basically and ultimately rests.

Theological Models for Administration

To seek proficiency as a pastoral administrator is a valid need and goal. To do so means to borrow liberally from a fund of knowledge outside of theology. In fact, today's pastor does such borrowing often in order to achieve functional competence in a variety of areas. The danger is that the absorption of such knowledge is done without theological filtering. For administrative proficiency alone must never be the goal. Rather the goal should be the enhancement and enrichment of ministry through better pastoral administration. To accomplish this, it is necessary that we look for theological models or biblical images to deepen our concepts of pastoral administration. What follows is an attempt to present some models and images that may be helpful in this process.

The Pastoral Administrator as King, Prophet, and Priest

Paul Tillich wrote that the church enters society in three ways: by interpenetration (the priestly), by critical judgment (the prophetic), and by political establishment (the kingly).[3] Pastoral administration is a blend of all three role models. The *king* exercises authority, uses power. At best, the king walks a tightrope between the abuse of power, which can result in tyranny, and the aversion of power, which can result in chaos. The administrator ought always to be ambivalent about power. Structures are needed to provide stability, but can become oppressive if perpetuated for their own sake. Flexibility enhances creativity, but without order it can provide license for irresponsibility.[4] The *prophet* critically assesses how the hospital makes decisions, formulates policy, treats people, establishes values. The prophet walks a similar tightrope between criticism and loyalty, recognizing that merely to mirror the dominant values of the hospital is political expediency, whereas to criticize incessantly runs the risk of impairing one's administrative effectiveness. The *priest* cares for individuals within the institution, and reaches out to the "victims" of that bureaucracy while, at the same time, being part of the power structure of that bureaucracy. The priest walks another tightrope between concern for the individual and for the organization. Both are important. Individuality is meaningless apart from community; but community is oppressive without individuality.[5] The priest also recognizes the subversive potential in both: organizations can exploit and depersonalize individuals by forcing them to sacrifice their wants and needs to the corporate good; individuals can seek to control organizations through their own narcissism and selfishness.

While these three role models do not provide solutions to all administrative problems, they do provide a much needed perspective on those tasks, as well as a corrective and a balance by acknowledging the often ambiguous claims placed upon the pastoral administrator to be king, prophet, and priest.

The Pastoral Administrator as Steward

The Scriptures repeatedly remind us that the things of this world are ours only as custodians. We can selfishly squander these resources, as did the dishonest steward in Luke 16:1–9, or we can fail to use them wisely, as did the servant in Matthew 25:14-30. In the midst of administrative decisions that impact the lives of both individuals and institutions, it is sobering to remind ourselves that we are managers, not owners; that these personal and material resources are God's, not ours.

In the New Testament descriptions of stewardship, some distinct qualifications emerge:

> *Shrewdness.* Jesus, through the swindled master, commends the dishonest steward for his prudence: "For the sons of this world are wiser (shrewder) in their own generation than the sons of light" (Luke 16:8).

> *Courage.* In the Parable of the Talents, Jesus reprimands the servant with one talent, not for his impoverishment but for his fear, which caused him to bury his talent rather than to employ it. (Matt 25:14-30).

> *Trustworthiness.* In describing servants of Christ as "stewards of the mysteries of God," Paul warns that one thing is required of stewards: "That they be found trustworthy" (1 Cor 4:2).

> *Selflessness.* "As each has received a gift," Peter admonishes, "above all hold unfailing your love for one another, since love covers a multitude of sins" (1 Pet 4:8).

The Pastoral Administrator as Sinner

As one takes seriously the profound and perverse effects of sin in individuals and in corporations, one can easily grow cynical. Yet better to be a realistic cynic than a naive enthusiast. As Luther once said: "The greatest sin is the pretense that we have no sin." Reinhold Niebuhr put it more strongly: "What is lacking among moralists is an understanding of the brutal character of the behavior of all human collectives and the power of self-interest and collective egoism in all intergroup relations."[6] He continued: "They [moralists] do not see that the limitations of the human imagination, the easy subservience of reason to prejudice and passion, and the consequent persistence of irrational egoism, particularly in group behavior, make social conflict an inevitability in human history, probably to its very end."[7] He concluded his grim analysis of the human situation: "Whatever increase in social intelligence and moral goodwill may be achieved in human history, may serve to mitigate the brutalities of social conflict, they cannot abolish the conflict itself."[8]

Saint Augustine felt that the individual and more particularly society are too involved in the sins of the earth to be capable of salvation in a moral sense.[9] He stated: "The city of this world is 'a compact of injustice,' its ruler is the devil and its place is secured by strife."[10]

Indeed, these are disparaging views that are not totally mitigated by the cross of Christ. That event turned defeat into victory and prophesied the day when love would be triumphant in the world. But the triumph will have to come through the intervention of God; the moral resources of men and women will never be sufficient to guarantee it. While the recognition of sin's perversity may appear devastating for any human enterprise, its admission may render the pastoral administrator less immobilized by idealism. Perfectionism can be psychologically and morally inhibiting. One who waits for the perfect moment to implement the perfect solution will wait a lifetime.

The admission of self-interest in all individual and corporate decisions ought to make us more modest about any plan or proposal. It ought to make us suspicious of any plan or proposal that unambiguously claims for itself absolute rightness. Indeed, to speak of absolutes in this way is to diminish the radical nature of sin.

Yet the good pastoral administrator recognizes that it is in this imperfect world that we must live our lives and exercise our stewardship. In so doing, it is necessary to explore carefully the spectrum of appropriate alternatives in any decision. To say that every situation is ambiguous, to admit to the reality of self-interest in every decision, is not to suggest that all decisions are appropriate or that all appropriate decisions are equally appropriate. Choices must be made, even with the full admission that no choice is without perversion and risk, that no choice is absolutely right. A pastoral administrator who acknowledges the awful power of sin lives always on the edge of preferred options.

The Pastoral Administrator as a Mortal among Mortals

Power and control can foster bizarre illusions. Long-range planning can feed the myth of perpetuity. One of my most humbling moments as a pastoral administrator comes each year when I clean out my file cabinet. It is then I discover the mortality of administration. How quickly memos and policies and position papers become outdated. How important they seemed at the time and how passionately I pursued their completion. Now they are dumped into the rubbish and duly forgotten.

Pastoral administrators, immersed in their daily tasks and assignments, ought to regularly remind themselves that "these too shall one day pass away." Unless we accept death (as individuals and institutions), which is our destiny, we do not live life to the fullest.[11] To affirm any structure without seeing its transiency is profane, yet on the other hand, to treat such with disdain because of its temporalness is irresponsible. To regard what is mortal as immortal is idolatrous; yet to disparage what is mortal simply because it is mortal is poor stewardship.

The Pastoral Administrator as a Priest among Priests

The call of the pastoral administrator to ministry is a spiritual gift, but it is not the only gift recognized in the Bible. A rich contribution of the Protestant Reformation was the recovery of the priestly role of all people, ordained and not, the recovery of "vocation" as God's call to all to be conformed to the mind of Christ. Job, family, society are but areas where that vocation, or calling, is lived out, hence, it follows that there is an essential democracy in God's kingdom. Each person has direct access to God; each has personal responsibility before him.

Though society confers privileges and differential through its rank and wage structures, the pastoral administrator must beware lest economic necessity be confused with reality. In God's eyes, no job or position is worth more than another, because no person is worth more than another. It is not the inherent nature of work that makes a worker important or makes work holy; rather, it is holy and committed people who make work sacred and important.

Through administration the pastor can validate this rich concept of vocation and encourage people to do well what they are doing. Such encouragements are more readily validated when the pastor's leadership encourages personal growth, not subservience; creativity, not conformity; mutuality, not autocracy. The priesthood of all believers provides a rationale for leadership that is essentially democratic and participatory.

The Pastoral Administrator as a Servant

One of the most meaningful and dramatic episodes in the life of Christ came on the eve of his death, in what was to be his last formal meeting with the disciples (John 13). Jesus girded himself with a towel, took a basin, knelt, and washed the disciples' feet. If ever we who administer need a model for leadership, there it is with Jesus at the disciples' feet. Power is subordinated to service; authority cloaked by humility. The managerial tools are not ROIs (return on investment), MBOs (management by objective), LISs (labor information statistics), or PFRs (project feasibility reports) but a towel and a basin of water—instruments of service.

The Pastoral Administrator as Redeemed

The chaplain's administrative decisions are terribly important with regard to the life of the hospital. Therefore they ought to be made carefully. They do impact the lives of others. However, those decisions are relatively insignificant with regard to anyone's ultimate destiny. For we are saved not by our moral rightness or by our administrative preciseness, but by God's mercy "which endures forever." Because the pastoral administrator knows something of God's redemptive action in the past, he or she dares to risk administrative actions in the present, with the conviction that such actions are done in the context of divine love and trust. For God trusts us. He trusts us with decisions and power — with his world. And though we at times are disloyal and incompetent, the gift of his trust remains.

NOTES

1. James Gustafson, "Political Images of the Ministry," *The Church, The University and Social Policy: The Danforth Study of Campus Ministries*, vol. 2, ed. Kenneth Underwood (Connecticut: Wesleyan University, 1968), p. 251.

2. Ibid., p. 251.

3. Paul Tillich, *Systematic Theology*, vol. 3 (Chicago: University of Chicago Press, 1963), p. 30.

4. Charles E. Hall, Jr., "Administrator as Juggler: The Paradoxical Nature of Life," *Cura Animarum*, The Association of Mental Health Clergy 36, no. 1 (May 1984): 34.

5. Ibid., p. 36.

6. Reinhold Neibuhr, *Moral Man and Immoral Society* (New York: Charles Scribner's Son, 1960), p. xx.

7. Ibid.

8. Ibid., p. xxiii.

9. Augustine, *The City of God*, as found in Niebuhr, *Moral Man*, p. 70.

10. Ibid.

11. Hall, "Administrator as Juggler," p. 38.

16

The Chaplain and
the Crisis in Ethics

KENNETH VAUX

"A New Theory of Biology" was the title of the paper which Mustapha Mond had just finished reading. He sat for some time, meditatively frowning, then picked up his pen and wrote across the title page, "The author's mathematical treatment of the conception of purpose is novel and highly ingenious, but heretical and, so far as the present social order is concerned, dangerous and potentially subversive. Not to be Published."[1]

The hospital board meeting was called to order. The chaplain offered the invocation. The first item on the agenda was a policy recommendation from the finance committee which ordered that Green Card (public welfare) patients not be admitted but be referred to the county hospital. The chairman claimed that the hospital had either to turn away charity patients or face a financial crisis. After reminding the chaplain that pastoral care's budget would be in jeopardy if such a fiscal crisis ensued, the chaplain was asked if there were any "religious" or "spiritual" considerations bearing on this contemplated policy.

"Don't bug me, chaplain," the young man cried, "I know what's going through your mind." The patient had AIDS (acquired immune deficiency syndrome). The chaplain knew that this serious, often lethal, disease was epidemic among homosexual persons. With guilt and shame compounding the very serious sickness, should the chaplain follow the inclination to offer an opportunity for confession and moral restitution, or should these hangups (moral sensibilities of patient and pastor) be repressed?

As soon as the chaplain entered the room the patient said, "Close the door, reverend. Tell me," he pleaded, "do I have cancer, am I going to die? My doctor won't tell me." The chaplain knew from a staff conference the week before that malignancy with a terminal diagnosis was present. What should the chaplain say?

To set the stage for discussion of the moral challenges and opportunities of the clinical ministry, I have chosen Aldous Huxley's biting rhetoric and three clinical-pastoral scenarios, each involving an ethical issue. The first case study concerns public morality or social ethics; the second, interpersonal concerns or interactional ethics; the third entails personal moral attitudes and choices. In addition to raising issues of particular moral dynamics, each case also calls attention to the fact that these pastoral dilemmas symbolize an intellectual and ethical crisis facing the broader culture.

To be a minister today is to find oneself caught up in an unenviable yet inevitable crisis. The clergy person symbolically embodies the spiritual and moral vitality and malaise of our time. Because of the disbelief and moral hesitancy of our particular age, the chaplain, or any minister who labors at a secular frontier, becomes a lightning rod which seems to draw down to earth's ground all the violent furies of heaven. This essay will examine the chaplain's function as a cobeliever with patients, families, and health professionals and as moral activist, prophet, advocate, and counselor.

Our generation is one that yearns to believe, that is, to have faith, hope, and love. It is also a generation that finds belief hard to come by. Faith traditions are no longer palpable and convincing. Onto this stage wanders the chaplain, embodying a religious world view, a strange compound of fancy and nostalgia, truth and wisdom. Though the chaplain's presence seems out of joint with our times, it still brings a comic delight and, more importantly, a haunting sense of judgment and possibility to our world.

While the chaplain is primarily an actor as opposed to a theoretician in the continuum stretching from pure theory to pure praxis, nevertheless ideas and convictions — a frame of reference, if you will — are betrayed and conveyed by all human living activity. In a certain sense, thinking discloses our beliefs (presuppositions, prejudices, epistomology, hope) and our acts express our values. We will need, therefore, to examine both *the moral activity* and *the underlying fabric of belief* to assess the ethical dimension of clinical ministry in our time.

This chapter argues that the contemporary cultural crisis, a crisis of belief and value, is symbolized poignantly by the health care crisis. This biomedical symptom of the broader crisis in the civilization can be accounted for *by the failure of medicine and theology to sustain a spiritual vision and moral conviction about the direction and legitimacy of the health care enterprise.* This moral vacuum has created both medical and religious compensatory aberrations. Religio-medical movements (Christian Science) and faith-health cults (Faith Assembly) show us the need for, and point us in the direction of, a new spiritual and moral possibility.

This thesis is developed in three stages: first, by sketching the dimensions of the prevalent culture crisis of disbelief and amorality as this is expressed in the health care crisis; second, by suggesting the outlines of an emerging renovation, one scientific, humanistic, and faithful to our universal faith experience; third, by suggesting how this new synthesis might find pioneering expression in the moral functioning of the chaplain.

The Crisis of Belief and Its Bearing on the Human Ministeries of Health

In his book *The Social Transformation of American Medicine,* Harvard sociologist Paul Starr contends that the profound crisis affecting modern medicine entails not only a crescendo of incredulity on the part of laypersons in the enterprise of medicine but also a decrescendo in the profession's own sense of authority.[2] The book carefully documents the fact that behind every traumatic crisis in health care practice lies a crisis of belief, and intellectual crisis.

Our first hypothetical example of a chaplain's involvement in health care concerned social ethics: should the poor be excluded from health care provision? At root, this not uncommon case reflects a crisis of morality and belief, of medical ethics and religion. Our ability to care when it costs is found defective because the underlying conviction which generates obligation is unsure. "The trouble with ministry today," a concerned Catholic layman told me recently, "is that they think if they get a person three squares a day they've done the job." "People need the 'Bread of Life,' not just bread." This blunt phrase reflects the mood of our age in which religious belief and welfare provisions are torn apart.

A brief review of the history and characteristics of this crisis of both belief and praxis (theory and technique) in religion and medicine may be made as follows. Until the early modern period Western civilization believed and tried to live by a world view that has been called "the Elizabethan world picture."[3] This perspective saw reality on a continuum from fundamental matter to pure spirit or God. The world was a providentially ordered hierarchical universe thrown askew by human sin, yet being drawn graciously into paradisal restoration and newness through Christ's redemption. All perceived reality—the sensational world of nature, the insights of reason, and the revelations of truth, good, and beauty—mediated this divine drama. Everything that happened to individuals and nations was part of the providential scheme. At the center of the "chain of being" and "cosmic dance"[4] stood the supernal yet earthly creature: the human person. Torn between creation and Fall, that person aspired to God and eternity yet declined toward the world, flesh, and the devil. God, the soul, and immortality, salvation and damnation, were the pervasive facts of existence. From the dawn of the Christian era until the nineteenth century this was the story that animated people's beliefs and actions.

This traditional Western or biblical-classical philosophy of the world and human existence also carried a specific theology of human life, health, and death. Because its source, destiny, and grounding were beyond this world, human health and life possessed ultimate dignity and sacrosanctity, but was to be the object only of penultimate and transient devotion. In *Hamlet* and *King Lear*, Shakespeare expresses the classical theology of death that the Hebrew Scripture, Plato, the Alexandrian Jews, and Augustine had formulated for Christian civilization. Ethical choices at the point of death were made in the light of this confidence that God stood near to receive one's life and that this life was not "all there is," nor did death mean extinction. Moral guidance and moral sustenance in the throes of death took on very distinct meanings. "Vex not his ghost," writes Shakespeare, "let him pass! He hates him that would upon the rock of this rough world stretch him out longer."[5]

But even Elizabethans began to see this world view fracture and collapse. Puritan scholars of the seventeenth century began to demand empirical verification to establish truth, refusing to accept Aristotelian, Galenic, or Thomistic theory as the *axis veritas* from which facts were deduced. Later generations would see the final demise of the great chain of being. Now the demarcation between lifeless and living, between energy and matter, appeared arbitrary. Science disclosed the cosmos whirling within the single cell and the atom. The microcosm disclosed its affinity to the macrocosm. God, the soul, and immortality, were now *qualities of faith, not objects of knowledge.*

Medieval cosmology also portrayed and conveyed a moral position.

Heaven and hell were enacted in the person's soul and conscience in the dynamics of salvation and damnation, grace and sin. If the art, literature, and architecture of a civilization are indicative of its ethos, this world view shaped the character of great and small, rich and poor. People thought of themselves as moral agents, addressed by a moral law, accountable to the will of an omnipotent deity, subject to present and eternal happiness or everlasting pain and sadness, depending on the state of one's soul. Destiny hinged on rightness, that is, upon moral justification and action.

While the actual quantum and intensity of human good and evil probably did not change greatly with the collapse of the biblical-classical world view, the framing context with its defining and motivating power was now vastly diminished.

The demise of traditional Western faith and love reached its intellectual epitome with the enthronement of reason in the midst of Notre Dame, the symbol of medieval Christendom. On through the nineteenth century, accompanying moral degradation withheld its full fury until the twentieth when science joined technology and totalitarian politics to devastate the human fabric of civilization as never before in history.

Health care, traditionally a correlate of salvation (*salve*) and an expression of religious care, *now became a function of scientific technology.* Human science since Darwin followed no other design than evolution; the French biochemist Jacques Monod has shown that biology unfolds by chance and mutation and not by necessity or purpose. As the traditional world view collapsed, modern medicine began to build itself upon this new theoretical foundation. Guiding values no longer flowed from theological purpose but from economic and political imperative. Just as theoretical physics yielded atomic warfare and caused Robert Oppenheimer to sadly muse that "what was technically sweet became irresistible," so biomedicine followed the same pattern. What could be done was done inevitably, without asking whether it should be done.

We now live in the age of patenting life, determining offspring by amniocentesis and sex-selection, controlling the mind through chemicals, electrodes, and surgery, and defying mortality by transplanting organs and maintaining terminal life-supports. This intellectual and moral revolution takes place in the modern hospital, the hostel created for the most part by faith-inspired compassion and the continuing setting of religious-clinical ministry.

In this world of sophisticated technique and diminished belief, the *moral sense remains even though the explanatory system has vanished.*

The main expression of theological amnesia today is humanistic existentialism. Perhaps the French existentialists were correct that the vestige of Judeo-Christian morality was just the smile of a Cheshire cat that lingered even though the cat was gone. If their claim was correct, then anything goes in the moral sphere. If God were nonexistent what claim could be made that war, violence, torture, and deception were wrong? Some believers attempted to construct an ethical framework upon some existential base such as Kierkegaard or Bultmann, which did not attempt to retain a pre-Copernican theological cosmology but distilled the essence of a gospel of subjective faith and a radical morality.

Most chaplains have adopted this compensation and find themselves existentialists. A central feature of the litany of Clinical Pastoral Education is to disavow thought and avoid the systematic formulation and evaluation of convictions. In the supervisory process, the chaplain is asked how he or she "feels." "What is really going on?" "You had your time of mental gymnastics and gesticulations in seminary," the C.P.E. student is instructed. "Now let's get down to where people really are." To alter a phrase of Marx, most chaplains would claim that "the philosophers seem to understand reality, we seek to clarify it." Philosophy in the analytic tradition concentrates more on language analysis than on normative ethics or metaphysics. Similarly, *the chaplain often avoids the rigors of belief in a post-Christian age by concentrating on caring, not asking why or to what end.*

I have argued in this first section that we find ourselves amidst a crisis of care—existential care. I contend that care for its own sake ceases to be care. Though a courageous gesture in a world stripped of belief, this care lacks staying power, continuity, and purpose. Ministry entails three modes of care: *soul care, moral guidance,* and *consolation.* By definition, each of these dimensions of care is pointless and impotent when torn from its enveloping belief structure.

It is not difficult to understand how we came to our present position. Love became moralistic, often pragmatic. Certainly, it was corrupt to offer counseling in order to save a soul when that caring did not flow from a heart of love. But now to offer counsel apart from some image of human wholeness or some dynamic of healing (salvation) is equally dangerous. The ethical life requires an undergirding theology. Moral direction implies a pattern of life that serves as normative standard. What of consolation? When someone dies most can only express sorrow. Though the words are tender and appreciated, they fail to console—only a faith in life in the face of death suffices.

Similarly, medical care revolves around three pivotal ministrations: *palpation or laying on of hands; exorcism or removing a toxic or noxious source of sickness; and conversation or therapy of the word.* Doctors in our day have trouble enacting these ministries not only because technology, (e.g., visualization, surgery, and specific therapy and diagnostic technology) is rendering them obsolete, but because the context of belief that once validated these symbolic expressions no longer animates many physicians. Medicine is becoming more and more a spectrum of impersonal technical transactions where diagnostic and therapeutic direction is given by scientific instrumentation. All the while, medical practice becomes sadder and more boring and the society becomes sicker. But denial and doubt, the spiritual malaise of our time, is not ennobling or convincing.

It appears that we could believe in reality as God given and directed if we knew less or if we knew more. Our present modicum of knowledge is enough to repudiate traditional belief and morality, but we suspect that if we knew more, for example, about cell biology, cosmology, or the human person, we might be redirected toward belief. When his gravely ill daughter began to recover, out of grateful delight Sigmund Freud threw his slipper against the wall intentionally breaking a valuable marble Venus from his priceless collection of antiquities. He later interpreted this as a sacrificial act:

> We ... or our primitive forefathers ... once believed that these possibilities (superstitions) were realities; and were convinced that they actually happened. Nowadays we no longer believe in them, we have surmounted these modes of thought, but we do not feel quite sure of our beliefs; and the old ones still exist within us ready to seize upon any confirmation. As soon as something actually happens in our lives which seems to confirm the old discarded beliefs we get a feeling of the uncanny.[6]

Though the healing enterprise and the religious ministry, as a dimension of that enterprise, now waiver for lack of a guiding purpose, there are premonitions even among the most scientific and skeptical of a new perception of reality. We are now experiencing not only a renovation of a former synthesis but, in some sense, a new frontier. This "new being," as Tillich would call it, moves our understanding of the moral posture of the clinical minister to another level. This new perception is not a regression to superstition as Freud might contend but a progression to greater scientific and humanistic insight.

The New Ethos Where Belief
and Morality Is Again Possible

Malinowski and other anthropologists have shown the close affinity between science and magic. Magic is the primitive attempt to discern the energy which animates natural process in order to bring it under control. Magic/science appears on a spectrum from fallacious understanding and nonefficacious manipulation (bleeding for smallpox) to very sophisticated theory and praxis (Einsteinian light theory and laser therapy). In the middle of the spectrum is theoretical half truth that gives deceptive signals of efficacy (Andrew Ivy's krebiozin, a cancer cure made from horse serum). Philosophers of science remind us that all irrational or rational theory only approximates, never fully captures, reality and that all manipulations are experimental (trial and error). In this sense, *magic and science are expressions of the same human ingenuity and creativity.*

The impact of this philosophical insight is far reaching. *It deals a lethal blow to the positivist distinction between fact and value. It establishes the relativity of science and enhances the possibility of faith.* The import of this new scientific insight (actually the contribution of the seventeenth-century English Puritans) is that *science and faith are not only compatible but are complementary approaches to reality.* The workings of nature and the movements of history (the dynamics of space and time) can now be perceived and responded to in a total world view, embracing both nature and supernature.

In a given period of history, the prevalent world view — especially as this shapes the aesthetic and ethical expression and perception of an age — determines the cultural awareness of the transcendent dimension; indeed, it determines the spiritual temper of that period. This sense of transcendence shapes belief and morality. *We are likely entering an era that will be remembered for the vitality of its science and vibrancy of its faith.* Indeed, it may be recalled not only as an age of belief but an age of goodness. This last assertion is made with great reservation given the pervasive materialism, hedonism, selfishness, and general destructiveness that we find everywhere. *But it can be argued that never before in history has the sense of the worth of the person and the advocacy of human rights been so intense.* The fact that abrogations of values and rights are so keenly felt may indeed provide evidence of this heightened sensitivity.

The import of this different way of experiencing reality upon the moral quality of clinical ministry now comes into focus. The way we view natural process gives rise to our notions of cause and effect. Our evaluation of why and how things happen the way they do in turn determines our views of freedom and responsibility.

Our second opening scenario dealt with the all-too-real scourge of our time, AIDS among homosexual men. The resurfacing of moral abhorrence and that cynical you-get-what-you-deserve attitude causes even considerate persons to ponder again themes such as "the wrath of God" or nature's retributive feedback cycle: "reaping what we sow." But, the religious perspective releases persons from a moral view based on natural necessity, determinism, or a punitive deity. (The latter attribution is always an extrapolation from nature's harsh retribution.) Grace, not inevitability, comes into play when beliefs of creation and fall chasten the concept of nature. There is brokenness, disorientation, and pain at the very heart of reality in the biblical view. Homosexuality is an excellent phenomenon to understand this fall within creation, of brokenness with health, of limitation within possibility. The best biological, psychological, and sociological research at present seems to point to the fact that homosexuality is a quality deeply enmeshed in human nature, one not completely attributable to sin or social determinism.

If, as the "at-once-new" and "very old" world view becomes ours, physical reality then is recognized as transparent to spiritual; preternal activity shines through the natural; and nature is seen as vibrant with grace. In the area of AIDS and homosexuality this means that forgiveness, transformation, and care, not judgment, inevitability, and contempt, are the order of the day. The opposite posture has most often prevailed in medicine and ministry. Plato reports in his *Republic*, "When intemperance and disease multiply in a State, halls of justice and medicine are always being opened; and the arts of doctor and lawyer give themselves airs . . . the physicians of old . . . would have nothing to do with unhealthy and intemperate subjects . . . the art of medicine was not designed for their good."[7]

At this point we do not know the cause of AIDS. We can say that homosexual activity among men is the cause. But in some countries, where we may assume homosexuality is practiced, there is no reported occurrence of the disease. Perhaps it is some specific viral or bacterial agent. Causality is probed by asking why and how this has happened. This causal question takes us to the heart of human ethics. "Be sure your sin will find you out," counsels the Hebrew Scripture. Does God, through the agency of beneficent and punitive will, bestow health (longevity, children, well-being) or illness? Does a moral law infuse nature, rendering its effect without respect to persons? Theological science has always held that God is both prime cause and the guiding direction of ongoing process. God is the author of cosmic activity and of historical events, and of human destiny (life and death).

If this faith and hope is valid, then human interaction can be viewed in a new light. At least three implications seem clear: first, persons are responsible for their actions before God alone. While we are not to lead others into evil but positively to encourage one another in the good, we are not accountable for the actions of others. Second, since purpose not chance governs human affairs, we are responsible for our life and each event is filled with redemptive meaning. Finally, grace, that is, freedom, possibility, and forgiveness contour human affairs. We are not doomed to some inevitable genetic or sociologic fate.

The chaplain is the mediator of, and witness to, this new moral reality. The world condemns; faith forgives, heals, and saves. For this reason the chaplain is often viewed as a trouble maker. Hospitals often become agencies of accounting, regularity, and bureaucracy rather than places where gracious spontaneity can flourish. The institution is committed to efficiency, profit-making, and uniformity. From the food services to the dispensing of medications and visiting hours everything must follow the prescribed protocol. The chaplain will often be found bucking this system.

We have argued that a new science makes possible a new theology that, in turn, creates a new ethical possibility. In this new understanding moral guidance and moral vision are again possible. The new science renders the amorality and antimorality of the nineteenth century and the early positivistic decades of the twentieth century obsolete. Amoralism contends that all values are culturally relative and that one ethic is as good as another. There are no normative criteria by which to judge values. While the new world picture does not allow for a single univocal normative standard that obliterates all variety and permutation in belief and value, *it does give new credence and moral power to consensual beliefs and to the insights of various value traditions.*

Is there a pattern for the healthy life-style? Is there a normative ideal to guide human sexuality, marriage, and human interrelations? Yes, it must now be argued. Features of the normatively human can be discerned. Moral ideals and guidelines for behavior can be postulated and defended. The moral option is not only possible, it is an essential ingredient of the fully human life. To deny this feature of existence is to reduce life to the subhuman. *It is now intellectually possible to affirm miracles, the sanctity of human life, and the existence of the soul.* Immortality and the moral nature of human life are again possible.

The chaplain therefore brings into concrete clinical and institutional decisions a vision of human life that renders judgment to any dehumanization or trivialization of persons, all the while advocating a positive picture of what human life could be and is meant to be.

Perhaps the major way that the chaplain needs to disturb the hospital system because of this new reality is to begin to minister to the institution, the staff, the administration, in addition to patients and their families. To concentrate care only on individuals who are hurting when the institution contributes in part to that malaise is foolish. The chaplain must also, always challenge the admonition to confine ministry to a "spiritual" box. "Stick to the spiritual needs of the patient, do not meddle in the secular affairs of peoples' lives." Following this mischievous counsel has been the demise of many ministries. We are to understand and help people in the wholeness of their lives not just some alleged sacrosanct part. On the other hand, we are to be authentically religious, not becoming two-bit psychiatrists or social workers by ingrafting those intellectual structures and practical therapies onto our own work.

Above, I argued that the new scientific world picture reintroduces providence and possibility back into our cosmos. *The chaplain therefore is both the reminder of a dying world and the harbinger of the new.* Here, I have shown that the new world picture fundamentally alters the dynamics of the moral life; replacing guilt with grace as the preeminent virtue. Now, I will contend that the character of moral action in ministry in this new day is one of *candor* and *consolation.*

Ethics as Care and the Requirements of Candor and Comfort

Don Browning of the University of Chicago, one of our most insightful pastoral theologians, has argued that "pastoral theology should rediscover itself as a dimension of theological or religious ethics. It is the primary task of pastoral theology to bring together theological ethics and the social sciences to articulate a normative vision of the human cycle."[8] Browning has correctly argued that the chaplain is foremost a theologian and that the crucial theological task of ministry, especially clinical ministry, is ethics. He has also pointed to the central task of practical theology as that of correlating religious experience with insight from the human sciences. The wisdom we are receiving today from ethology, biology, psychology, and the other human sciences is a truth about the transience and fragility of human existence and of the liberating power of personal hope and interhuman concern. I shall briefly summarize these insights and reflect on their significance for the moral activity of the chaplain.

The human sciences, ranging from genetics to social psychology, are pointing to the marvelous individuality and uniqueness of persons, the power of cultural images and values on shaping perceptions and behaviors, the pervasive fragility and interdependence of human persons and the power of trust, hope, and care to release human power so that even finitude and death is stripped of its terror.

The human sciences, especially genetics, human biology, and psychology are showing us the capacity for self-transcendence that inheres in every person. Not only do human beings carry a profound genetic heritage and adaptive capacity, but this cultural memory and preservation instinct provokes a power of self-relation that resembles altruism. This new knowledge about the intrapsychic and interself relation gives new credence to Kierkegaard's notion of the human person as transcendent to ultimate power, to the being of God. The principal evidence of this characteristic is the capacity of persons for shame and sympathy—primitive intrinsic expressions of the inescapable moral quality of human existence.

The most astonishing insight that modern science has yielded on human persons is the affirmation of ancient wisdom, which was expressed in the phrase, "strength is perfected in weakness." *Human beings are extremely vulnerable physically and emotionally but they achieve awesome strength in effective interchange with the physical environment and in the healing and supportive* (even vexing) *reciprocity with their fellows.* "Happy are the meek," spoke Jesus in the Sermon on the Mount. "They shall inherit the earth." In brokenness one finds wholeness; in self-surrender, self-discovery; in death, life.

Pierre Teilhard de Chardin has argued that the evolution of human species within the cosmos has created a highly intelligent and technically powerful creature at once profoundly sensitive to and vulnerable to suffering. *The development of highly myelinated frontal cortex in human persons has greatly enhanced intelligence but at the same time has rendered hopes, disappointments, joys, and agonies more acute.*

Human knowledge about the neural and emotional apparatus of persons also indicates that this vulnerability renders the person uniquely capable of interrelation, interdependence, and the power to mutually support and inspire.

Theological knowledge today is moving along the same axis. No longer is the human being the dominating lord of the cosmos against the pale background of a subservient environment. Humans are creatures of God, dependent for self-realization on his grace and given over to the tasks of justice and love as requirements of wholeness in existence. Armed with this twofold knowledge from science and faith, the chaplain is called to a moral ministry of sympathy, candor, and consolation.

The chaplain stands by the patient not so much with answers, and certainly not with judgment or condemnation, *but with profound identification*. Just as the woman who has undergone a mastectomy offers the deepest understanding to a new mastectomy patient, so the chaplain is a person who seeks to die into life, to be chastened in suffering, to offer cohumanity and companionship. In this posture candor is crucial.

Our third pastoral vignette had to do with a cancer patient who wanted to know the truth. There is no room for deception, cajoling, and lying. We bring truth to one another because love can only be found in truth and love casts out fear.

Finally, consolation is that gentle staying care that liberates joy from suffering, and life from dying. It remains the chaplain's principal art.

In this paper we have contended that a traditional world view that once undergirded belief and moral action has yielded to a new scientific and religious understanding. This constitutes a different framework for moral living which activates a pastoral style of care, candor, and consolation. The final word now is care in the face of finitude and death because these conceal salvation and life. In the film *An Officer and a Gentleman*, a young man, raised in the seedy environment of navy seaports by a drunken father, enters the rigorous discipline of naval pilot training and in the proces is liberated from meaninglessness and self-concentration to love and human care. The bondage of his past is shattered by the relentless demands of a sergeant, the genuine love of a simple seaport girl, and the absurd death of his first close friend.

The clinical ministry finds its setting amid the drama of birth, healing and life, suffering, pain and death. It is, if you will, the drama of damnation and salvation. Here, in Cicero's words, life's pretense is stripped away and we find ourselves "the dying caring for the dying." It is in this moral struggle that we receive life abundant.

NOTES

1. Aldous Huxley, *Brave New World* (London: Granado Press, 1931), p. 143.

2. Paul Starr, *The Social Transformation of American Medicine* (New York: Basic Books, 1982), p. 43.

3. E. M. W. Tillyard, *The Elizabethan World Picture* (London: Penguin Books, 1960), p. 43.

4. Ibid, p. 75.

5. *King Lear* V iii.

6. Sigmund Freud, "The Uncanny," *The Standard Edition of the Complete Psychological Works* (London: The Hogarth Press, 1953), pp. 244-48.

7. Plato, *The Republic*, trans. Benjamin Jowett (Cleveland: World, 1946), pp. 88, 92.

8. Don Browning (ed.), "Pastoral Theology in a Pluralistic Age," *Practical Theology* (New York: Harper & Row, 1983) p. 187.

17
The Chaplain as
Peripatetic Teacher

ARTHUR BICKEL and DAVID MIDDLETON

"The most universal and most appreciated role of Christian ministry through the ages has been teaching."[1]

Historically, teaching is at the core of our pastoral ministry. From the beginning of the Christian era teaching has been an integral part of pastoral ministry. The importance of teaching in the early church had its antecedents in the role of the rabbi in the Jewish community. Jesus was rabbi, or teacher, and his followers were disciples or learners.

As the disciples became apostles, they were commissioned to go and teach. Teaching became the primary mode of communication of the apostles, including Paul. This is not surprising for a movement that arose out of Judaism, which was rooted in the Torah or "teaching." The ability to teach was considered an essential qualification for pastoral leadership in the pastoral epistles (1 Tim 3:3).

The importance of teaching in ministry was reemphasized by the reformers as they valued biblical knowledge. In fact, the call for reformation came primarily from teaching clergy, the faculty at Wittenberg University. Calvin especially emphasized the teaching role in ministry and, to this day, Presbyterian pastors are officially ordained as "teaching elders."

In a 1956 study of Protestant pastors, Samuel Blizzard attempted to divide the work of the parish minister into six separate functions: (1) preacher, (2) pastor, (3) priest, (4) teacher, (5) organizer and (6) administrator.[2] He asked six hundred pastors to rank these functions in terms of their importance and to rank their own effectiveness in, and enjoyment of, them. It is interesting to note that they ranked teacher as fourth in importance and third in terms of their own effectiveness and enjoyment. However, teaching was assigned last place in the allotted use of time. These pastors claimed that teaching accounted for only one twentieth of their working time.[3]

The self-image and role of the pastor have certainly changed since this study in the mid-fifties and may have moved in the direction of greater appreciation for the role of teacher in ministry. In fact, in his first revision of *The Christian Pastor* in 1964, Wayne Oates said that "the minister's identity can be integrated most effectively around his (or her) role as teacher."[4] No doubt there is some difficulty in separating teaching as a function distinct from other functions. It may be seen as woven through all that we do. It is a thread running through the fabric of our ministry.

While there were no comparable studies of hospital chaplains, it may be assumed that we would envision our basic role in much the same way as our pastoral counterparts in the parish. There may well be differences in the allotment of time to different functions that would be demanded by the nature of the different settings in which we work. For example, it might be expected that hospital chaplains would spend far more time in pastoral visitation than parish clergy and less time in preaching. In fact, a recent survey of chaplains by the College of Chaplains of the American Protestant Hospital Association shows that teaching rated quite high in the use of time. This survey divided the roles of chaplains into twelve categories (each with subcategories), and asked respondents to indicate the average percent of time spent in each category. The categories were: (1) administrator, (2) advocate, (3) comforter, (4) consultant, (5) counselor, (6) liaison, (7) pastor, (8) prophet and ethicist, (9) sacramental leader, (10) teacher, (11) visitor of the sick, and (12) other. These categories are not discreet and the results are not very clear. However, teaching, with its subcategories of educator, theologian, and supervisor, was listed as taking 90 to 100 percent of the chaplain's time.[5] This survey helps to dispel any view that education constitutes a minor portion of the work of hospital chaplains.

A review of the annual special edition on pastoral care, *Bulletin of the American Protestant Hospital Association* (which publishes the workshop presentations by hospital chaplains), is an indication that chaplains are seriously applying themselves to the task of educating one another. Even though considerable time and energy appears to be devoted to educational tasks, there appears to be little that has been written about teaching and education as part of the chaplain's identity or role. In fact, we seem to have given relatively little attention to this in Clinical Pastoral Education that prepares clergy for institutional ministry. The reasons for this lack of attention to the role of chaplain as educator are not clear.

But the result has been a lack of appreciation for the teaching role of chaplains.

Some Misconceptions

One possible misconception is *that education is primarily, or even solely, the responsibility of chaplains who are designated or certified to be educators.* Some chaplaincy programs are divided between pastoral services and pastoral education. While this is administratively convenient, it may give the subtle impression that education is the specialized task of the chaplains in the educational section and not an important part of the work of those chaplains who are in the clinical or service area. Hence, education may be seen as the exclusive responsibility of those chaplains who are certified as clinical pastoral educators (C.P.E. chaplain supervisors).

In reality, most clinical or service chaplains are significantly involved in education at many levels. They are often involved in the education of parish pastors, laity, and other chaplains in a rich variety of ways. Even in Clinical Pastoral Education, service chaplains can make important contributions out of their clinical experience. They are important resources in the education of pastoral students. At our hospital we utilize clinical chaplains as coeducators in the supervision of one-year residents in Clinical Pastoral Education. This concept of multiple supervision involves a certified clinical pastoral educator (supervisor) who is responsible for the overall supervision of the student, including the peer group. Individual or clinical supervision of each resident student is done by a clinical chaplain who is considered a specialist on the unit to which the student is assigned. In other words, if the clinical assignment is on a pediatric unit the pediatric chaplain, who knows the unit best, becomes the individual supervisor whom we call "the clinical pastoral consultant." Clinical pastoral consultants may or may not be certified clinical pastoral educators. Their supervision work is integrated with, and coordinated by, the C.P.E. supervisor. This model of supervision is based on our appreciation of the educational contribution of the clinical chaplain and the conviction that this is an educational resource that should not be neglected. We believe that to do otherwise would be poor stewardship of our resources.

A closely related misconception is simply *a lack of appreciation of the teaching role as an important part of our ministry.* In pastoral education this may be seen as an emphasis on the development of counseling skills without a corresponding emphasis on teaching and educational skills. We are conversant with psychological theory, but not as aware of educational theory and the principles of learning.

This lack of appreciation for the place of education in the work of the minister is not confined to hospital chaplains. It seems to be shared with pastors generally. Seward Hiltner has suggested that, in spite of the emphasis on the teaching role of the minister in the New Testament and by the reformers, pastors have frequently failed to appreciate teaching as an important part of their task.[6] This neglect of the teaching role in ministry may be due to some deep seated ambivalence that is rooted in history. Hiltner suggests several reasons for this by saying that, "In spite of the emphasis placed by the *Protestant Reformers*, especially Calvin, upon the function of teaching, no image of the ministry as teaching — apart from preaching — has come down to us from that age."[7] One of the reasons suggested by Hiltner is that teaching became overidentified with the schools, even the church schools. Those who worked in the schools became identified as teachers and their work came to be viewed as another form of ministry. The ministry of teaching became separated from the overall work of the pastor. This separation of functions and the tendency toward specialization in ministry continues to affect us today.

Perhaps another misconception that hinders our full recognition of the educational work we do is *that view which sees education as only that which is done formally.* It is easy to fall into the trap of seeing as educational work only that which is programmed and scheduled. When one of the clinical chaplains on our staff was asked what kind of education he did, he replied that teaching patients and staff was what his ministry was about. It is true that most of the education we do is done informally, in the midst of situations, and not programmed, scheduled, or in a classroom.

Still another misconception that inhibits our claim to be educators is *that view which would limit our perception of our educational task to what we teach.* In other words, we are teaching only when we do it directly. However, we are providing a ministry of education when we recognize a need for learning and bring the learners and the educational resources together in an educational relationship. Our educational task is not limited to teaching. It is realized more fully in administering educational programs, relationships, and events.

Teaching is inherent in our role as pastors. It is influenced and enhanced by the special clinical settings in which we work. The hospital setting presents us with many educational needs and a variety of resources for addressing those needs. We also bring a unique combination of gifts and experience with which to address the educational needs in this setting.

More than most pastors, hospital chaplains are forced to seek correlations between theology and the behavioral sciences, between religious experience and the personal dynamics of believers. Because of their context, hospital chaplains also move between illness and healing. As Larry Holst put it, "The hospital chaplain walks between the world of religion and medicine, the Church and the hospital" (for a fuller development see chap. 2 above, "The Chaplain Between Worlds"). As educators we can bring the wisdom of religion and theology to bear some light on the world of medicine. We can also inform the theology and pastoral practice of others by interpreting the clinical setting and living experience we find there. In keeping with the original intent of Anton Boisen, the founder of C.P.E., we become the theologians of the "living human documents."

Finally, a common misconception occurs when we join society in *equating teaching with instruction, the imposing or imparting of information by an expert.* In such a view, learning is the accurate absorption of information that has been presented. To be sure, this is one form of education, one which we experienced in most of our schooling. There is, however, another form of educating which occurs, for instance, between a child and parent. This is not confined to the imparting of information, but includes challenge, encouragement, understanding, celebration, suggestion, invitation, and blessing of the learning process of the child. It is more child-centered learning than expert-centered learning.

Patients are learners before we ever meet them. Some are intense and vigorous learners and have been all their life. Some are passive learners, inclined to wait for learning to rap on their door. The etymology of the word *education* comes from the Latin *educare*, "to lead out." That is a very important function of the teaching chaplain, namely, to walk with the patient while the patient learns, tries to make sense of, finds new values, affirms old values, discovers, and gains insight into self. The function of the teaching chaplain in much patient care is best described as facilitating, enhancing, encouraging, and walking with the learner.

A New Image

If an image is needed to recover an appreciation for the place of teaching in pastoral ministry, perhaps it is to be found in "the peripatetic teachers" of the ancient world. "Peripatetic" comes from the Greek *peripatetikos*, which is a conjunction of two words, *peri*, "around," and *patein*, "to walk." It was used to describe Aristotle who walked around as he taught in the Lyceum. It implies an itinerant style of teaching that is done as one moves about or walks from place to place.

This image is certainly consistent with the ministry of Jesus, who roamed about the countryside and into the villages and cities with the Twelve, teaching them, the other disciples, and other followers. He taught in the synagogues, on the hillsides, at the beach, in boats, at a well, and at the city gates. He taught people wherever he encountered them. He responded to questions. He taught in the context where people lived and worked, celebrated and suffered, rejoiced and grieved. He taught through dialogue. He taught the estranged woman who came to the well in the noonday heat. He confronted the crowd that was ready to execute a woman caught in an adulterous relationship.

The hospital chaplain, perhaps more than anyone else engaged in pastoral ministry, has the opportunity to be a present day "peripatetic teacher." We work in an environment that demands on-the-spot immediate educational response. It is a setting that invites educational dialogue as we are being bombarded by theological questions. It is a context in which people, physicians and patients, nurses and families, are raising ultimate questions in relation to immediate circumstances of their lives. Questions about life, its value and meaning, the place of suffering, evil and the will of God are not mere academic questions in this context.

The chaplain frequently encounters a variety of such questions. Why do good people suffer? Does it do any good to pray? Should we consider a do-not-resuscitate order? They are not always questions. They may be bold challenges, debates, or subtle hints. They probe for the will of God, the meaning of life, the meaning of suffering, and guidelines for anguished moral decisions. More often than not our response is that of a teacher, helping others to seek wisdom and truth and to find their own integrity.

Four Crucial Attitudes

The hospital chaplain, a peripatetic teacher in formal and informal settings, teaches out of the ground of faith. And out of spiritual commitment the chaplain is challenged to assume certain attitudes as a teacher. We will look at four of those crucial attitudes: to teach (1) *with tentative* certainty, (2) *with a sense of mutuality*, (3) *with respect for the learner*, and (4) *with humble gratitude*.

Teach with Tentative Certainty

In order to teach, we have to have some convictions. The convictions we have are those formed in living, in working, in personal education, in reading, in relationship with fellow human beings and in relationship with God. Part of our motivation for entering the ministry originated with the realization that we have found, or have been found by, some truth in life that we have experienced as inspiring, helpful, enlightening, or saving. We were moved to share that inspiration and enlightenment. Theologically, this is the concept of witness originating with conviction.

At the same time, we have a crucial awareness that our insight, our awareness, our convictions are limited and may be erroneous, or misinformed. With the Apostle Paul we "know in part." We are human; creatures not Creator. And as we search for understanding, our convictions are sometimes altered, expanded, tentatively held or even discarded. Gordon Allport considered such heuristic duality (knowing but not knowing fully) a characteristic of religious maturity.[8] By the grace of God we continue to grow so we are people with some light to share, who at the same time have our problems with darkness.

It can be refreshingly helpful for a student, a patient, a colleague in the ministry to see our tentativeness, along with our convictions, our resilience with our firmness. This teaching stance is particularly evident when we walk with patients who are struggling with the mysteries of God's ways, asking questions for which there are no apparent, certain answers. In fact, it is probably true that the most important learning people gather from us is that they can hold to faith in the face of uncertainty and still live with hope, gratitude, and love. It is important for us to be open and supple so that the Holy Spirit can further enlighten us. It is equally vital that those whom we teach see our limits and our strengths lest we leave them with the impression that we have all the answers and that they should, too.

Teach with a Sense of Mutuality

This is a first principle of pastoral care suggested by Paul Tillich.[9] The Division of Pastoral Care at Lutheran General has a weekly staff meeting which includes a devotional meditation. The morning this copy was being written, one of our chaplains talked about how much she was learning from her child of three and a half years. Learning is mutual even between parent and child. It may be that God gave the teaching ministry to human beings and not angels because human ministers know what learning is about and out of their own learning can more readily join with fellow human learners. Teaching and learning in ministry are inseparable and simultaneous. How often, in ministering to patients, have we walked away from them with a sense of awe for their courageous faith, indomitable spirit, infectious appreciation for life and recovery, or their amazing capacity to care for others. We learn much from them.

As C.P.E. supervisors, some of us have fantasized beginning a C.P.E. program by sending students to see patients for two weeks, who will refrain from offering any ministry and concentrate on learning from patients what it means to be sick and hospitalized. One of the educational methods we have used in C.P.E. is to have a student bring a patient into a seminar. We contract explicitly with the patient — we do not want to teach anything but we want the patient to teach us what it means to be a patient, including what it means spiritually. We have done it often and consistently find patients willing to talk, even about their faith and relationship to God. Some patients who have been active in the church often say that they have never done that before and have found it very helpful. It appears that we are so busy in the church talking at and teaching folks that we have neither the time nor inclination to listen and learn from them. One of the most stimulating privileges we have as teaching chaplains is to learn while we teach — to grow, to change, to progress, because in giving we receive from those who receive our ministry of teaching.

Teach with Respect for the Learner

The inclination to be impersonal is never far away in a hospital. The problem of depersonalization lingers about in all phases of hospitals, including our ministry as teachers. It may sometimes work in reverse as patients overgeneralize in talking about "the typical doctor" or "all nurses." Sometimes we engage in that depersonalization in order to survive the agony. But the challenge remains to approach every human being with reverent respect as a creature of God. Behaviorally, this is the recognition that each person is a "thou" and that to relate to the other as an "it" is to violate that other's integrity. We teach creatures of God who are the crown of creation, created in the divine image. We are complex. Each of us is on a unique pilgrimage through the miseries and ecstasies of life. We have amazing spiritual capacities to grow, to endure, to hold by faith, to be creative, and to understand.

In Clinical Pastoral Education, the ever present yearning of students to learn, to better understand, to become more competent in ministry, to realize their potential is an awesome reality. We are not, first of all, students, patients, professional staff, clergy, or clients. We are first of all human beings who often in the process of learning and teaching invite each other into the holy ground that is our person: where we cherish values, experiences, and loved ones; where we struggle with our faults, our blindness, our sin; where we celebrate the capacity of our minds to comprehend and our spirits to grow. Our very best moments as ministering teachers occur when we approach the other person with a sense of deep respect.

Teach with Humble Gratitude

With education, training, and experience may come feelings of competition, superiority, and arrogance. We may come to see others as uninformed or ignorant, much in need of our teaching. We are more on track when we remember that we are still learners ourselves. All our knowledge and experience came to us because others passed it on to us. We were affirmed and challenged to grow by significant teachers, authors, and the people in our lives. Nothing that we know is original to us. It is all a gift. What is unique to us is our particular arrangement and variety of knowledge and experience. It is that uniqueness which adds a special variety to our own teaching and learning. To be valued as the teacher of others is a privilege, and it is good for us to remember that by letting us be learners others gave us the opportunity to walk with them as they grew. They are worthy of our gratitude.

The Benefits of Education

Commitment to the education function of pastoral care represents investment of time, energy, and money. It is appropriate to ask what kind of return, what kind of benefit, is realized from that commitment. In our opinion, the most important benefits come as a result of what we earlier described as the peripatetic teaching ministry of the chaplain.

There are other, lesser but important benefits. We speak now primarily of benefits we have seen at our hospital as a result of the more formal, structured forms of education with community clergy and laity and Clinical Pastoral Education students. The various educational structures include one or two day seminars, a series of courses over several weeks, full time C.P.E. programs and programs for lay people interested in developing more competence in visiting the sick and shut-ins.

The chaplain as an educator stands in an important position in the relationship of the hospital to the larger community. Because of the chaplains' relationship to the hospital and to the religious community and institutions, there is a tremendous opportunity to do some bridging between the two. The church and clergy often have educational needs that can be addressed by the hospital's resources. Also, there are resources beyond the hospital that may be helpful in that setting. The chaplain is often in a unique position to bring learners and resources together in a creative educational relationship. This kind of educational relationship between hospital and religious community helps to develop a more healthy sense of community and to foster more understanding, as it also heightens the hospital's visibility in the community. Further, it can bridge misunderstandings that may develop between a hospital and that community.

A related benefit is that educational programs offered to the religious community help to develop more informed members of its caring team. The many orientation programs that hospitals provide for community clergy, and the ongoing seminars designed to assist them in visiting and understanding their hospitalized parishioners, are good examples. In our hospital there have also been programs to train and orient Roman Catholic lay persons who distribute communion to Catholic patients. This program has been strengthened and enhanced through a sound educational approach.

One very apparent benefit of educational efforts is the multiplication of resources. For instance, one clinical pastoral educator can work with as many as six students, which means that six people are spending a major portion of their time seeing patients. The number of hospitals with volunteer pastoral care staffs have grown significantly in the past few years. These function best when trained and organized by a full-time chaplain or chaplains. These volunteer chaplains sometimes number thirty to forty in a single institution. They provide considerable time and service to the hospital by visiting patients, working through the night in emergency room ministry, or being available for on-call crises. In exchange, the hospital offers regular continuing education seminars, planned and arranged by the pastoral care staff. In this time of concern for cost effectiveness among health care institutions, the principle of multiplication of resources is a realistic factor supporting the educational functions of chaplains.

Another significant benefit of this type of education is the appreciation and support it demonstrates for community clergy and their congregations. Such programs are often seen by those clergy and their people as gestures of service and good will on the part of the hospital. A vital conclusion drawn by the clergy and congregations is that the hospital respects the importance of their faith, their relationship with God, in matters of sickness and health.

Another benefit we have become sensitive to in our hospital is that through our C.P.E. programs we have made major contributions to the national and international church, as well as the Jewish community. Our hospital opened its doors in 1959 with a one-year C.P.E. residency already established. Since that time there have been 470 students of all faiths in our accredited programs (varying in length from three months to two years). Among that number have been foreign students from Taiwan, Mexico, Finland, Norway, Sweden, Germany, New Guinea, Africa, Australia, Scotland, Canada, and the Philippines who have returned to serve in their native lands. Follow up studies of our past C.P.E. residents reveal that about 30 percent are presently serving as parish ministers and 70 percent are in institutional ministry or full-time counseling ministries. Especially for hospitals that owe their origins to the vision, commitment, and sacrifice of the religious community, this is a particularly satisfying benefit. The hospital thus, in turn, serves the church which was initially responsible for its coming into being.

An important benefit is that formal educational efforts usually result in personal satisfactions for the chaplains. In the language of management, the chaplain experiences more job satisfaction. The chaplains express appreciation for the variety that education affords. Chaplaincy is a narrow specialized ministry working with hospitalized patients. Formal educational efforts offer a welcome and stimulating change of pace for pastoral care staff.

In addition, the growth that occurs in students is often marked and immediate. They tend to be readily discernible to both learner and educator. In many other aspects of hospital ministry the results are less tangible and overtly gratifying. In our C.P.E. programs some of our chaplains who are specialists in clinical areas (e.g., coronary care or psychiatry) are involved in overseeing students, though they are not certified C.P.E. supervisors. They experience the satisfaction of sharing their expertise with students and, in turn, seeing the students grow in pastoral maturity and competency.

Last, education challenges the pastoral care staff. The inquisitive spirit of educational programs stimulates the teacher's own continued growth. The teaching chaplains are challenged to sharpen teaching skills as well as to stay informed and current in their own thinking and reading. Continual reexamination of their own ministry, along with the stimulation of educational ventures, helps to keep the chaplains relevant in their total ministry.

NOTES

1. Henri J.M. Nouwen, *Creative Ministry* (New York: Doubleday, 1971), p. 3.

2. Samuel Blizzard, "The Minister's Dilemma," *The Christian Century* (25 April 1956): 508–510. A fuller commentary on this may be found in Wayne Oates, n. 4 below.

3. Ibid.

4. Wayne Oates, *The Christian Pastor* (Philadelphia: Westminster Press, 1964), p. 108.

5. *The Tie*, newsletter of the College of Chaplains, American Protestant Hospital Association, 18 no. 5 (October 1982).

6. Seward Hiltner, *Ferment in the Ministry* (Nashville and New York: Abingdon Press, 1969), pp.86ff.

7. Ibid.

8. Gordon Allport, *The Individual and His Religion* (New York: MacMillan Co., 1959), p. 72ff.

9. Paul Tillich, "The Theology of Pastoral Care," *Pastoral Psychology* (October 1959): 21–26.

18

The Chaplain and Lay Ministry

FLORENCE FLYNN SMITHE

It was a warm summer evening in 1974 when my husband and I found ourselves and our nine-year-old son in the emergency room of Lutheran General Hospital. Tim had been struck in the face with a bat while playing softball. He was in a lot of pain, his face badly bruised and bleeding. We were all frightened and particularly concerned that he might have sustained a skull fracture.

While we anxiously awaited X-ray reports, we were visited, quite unexpectedly, by the emergency room chaplain. He introduced himself to us and we learned that this chaplain, serving patients of all faiths in a Lutheran hospital, shared our faith as Roman Catholics. It was a pleasant surprise.

The chaplain's presence was a source of great comfort for each one of us. We experienced him sharing deeply in our concern, particularly in the initial moments when the crisis was being evaluated. He listened carefully and sensitively and he prayed with us. When we were told that Tim's injury was not life threatening, he shared in our joy and thanksgiving.

Tim was admitted to pediatrics and scheduled for surgery to repair his broken nose. Although doctors reassured us that he would recover completely, we continued to feel our anxieties rise and our energy fall. A young man was one of the many hospital personnel who came to Tim's room. He introduced himself as the duty chaplain. He had been told of Tim's accident by a nurse and wanted to see how we all were doing. He communicated a special warmth and caring, even inquiring about our other children and Tim's grandparents. We learned at the conclusion of his visit that he was a student from Garrett Theological Seminary. He explained that his chaplaincy position was part of the course of study in Clinical Pastoral Education. His visit was surprising to us in several ways. First, we were experiencing the ministry of a Protestant seminarian and it did not feel invasive. His ministry felt very appropriate and very comforting. Until that moment, I had never considered the possibility that someone other than a Catholic priest could be the proper minister to our family. Second, we had no idea that a process for learning ministry existed outside of seminary walls.

Tim's surgery was successful, and following his recovery my husband and I talked about the new ministers who had been so significant to us during this crisis. As a result of that process another surprising thing happened. My husband suggested that I should apply for the Clinical Pastoral Education program. I was stunned by his suggestion. I had just expanded my understanding of ministry from priest to Protestant clergy and now he was suggesting that I, as a lay person, could be included.

The idea took several months to take hold; clearly I had heard the call to participate more fully in ministry. Time passed and I continued to flirt with this new challenge. One day I received a call from the hospital's blood bank. They needed a blood donor with my blood type immediately. At that moment, I knew that the day had come when I would respond to the other call.

As I lay quietly on the table in the blood bank, I believe I had a peak religious experience. Suddenly I was aware of a sense of awe and wonder and of being beyond myself. Something remarkable was happening. I felt profoundly aware of God's presence there and of the words "today will change the direction of my life and the life of lay women in the church." Later I remember feeling secretly embarrassed by the rather grandiose (and sexist) nature of the experience and yet, there it was. A sense of the Spirit guiding and urging me on my journey. I left the blood bank and found my way to the pastoral care office. I left there with some brochures and an application, a bit stunned by the rapid and profound sequence of the day's events.

A short time later, the acceptance of my application was received. From the moment of my acceptance into the program, personal concerns emerged. Thirty-four years old, a wife and mother of seven children under fifteen years of age, I had serious concern regarding my ability to "manage" it all. My husband promised to provide the support necessary, just as he had provided the initial call. Other questions quickly presented themselves when the program began. Most threatening of all was my personal identity crisis. Who me—a minister? Would I be accepted by the staff clergy? Would I be accepted by the patients ? It didn't take long for the answers to come. In part, they came through an early, meaningful encounter.

Marie, a forty-five-year-old cancer patient, was dying. Nurses caring for her expressed some special concerns to me. They were puzzled by her husband's instructions, "No one is to discuss the seriousness of her illness with her." He had also informed them that there would be no other visitors besides their immediate family.

Stopping in the doorway of Marie's room, I observed that she appeared to be sleeping. Her labored breathing was being assisted by an oxygen tube. Her right hand was stretched over a board to protect the intravenous needle that was giving her nourishment through a vein. Her thin body was covered lightly with a sheet. There were a few cards and flowers, signs of those persons who cared. Feelings of sadness and emptiness came over me as I looked on this scene of suffering and loneliness. Marie began to stir, and as our eyes met I approached her bedside. A gold and white plastic crucifix, a rosary, and a well-worn prayer book on the bedside table gave clear evidence of the patient's faith. Quietly, I explained to Marie that I was a lay chaplain and that I would be stopping by each day if that was all right with her. She nodded that it would be. "A priest is available if you would like to see him," I told her. She did not reply. Clearly, Marie was very weak and this factor combined with her husband's instructions regarding her condition would limit the scope of our verbal communication.

During our visits in the days that followed, we would simply be together. When Marie desired, we would pray one of the prayers marked with a holy card in her prayer book. One day, as I was reading a special prayer for healing, Marie opened her eyes and said, "He'd better hurry." I knew then that Marie knew that she was dying. Holding her hand tightly, I sensed in our presence and our touch that we were communicating deeply with one another.

The next morning nurses alerted me that Bill, her husband, had been called to the hospital during the night. It was only a matter of time. I found him staring out a window at the end of the hall. I explained that I was a lay chaplain and that I had come to know his wife during this hospitalization. His response came in a burst of anger. "And where are the priests now?" After a few moments he relaxed a little and began to explain his disappointment with the church. Two years ago, when they had first learned that Marie had cancer, Bill left word at their parish house for their pastor to visit Marie. No one came, even after a second call was made. That, Bill explained, was the beginning of their separation from the church. For whatever reason their pastor did not come, Bill and Marie felt rejected by the church and had broken their relationship with it at the time they needed it most.

At this point I sensed that my presence as a lay minister may have been of particular value as he struggled to express his anger toward God, the clergy, and the church. Bill was asking those painful questions: "Why this disease?" "Why now, when we have so much to live for?" He told me then of their life together, their hopes and dreams for the future. "She is all that matters to me," he said. "And now amidst so much suffering, I am going to lose her."

We sat quietly together and Bill was crying. After a little while I asked, "Do you think Marie might want to see a priest?" "No!" He replied firmly. "Then she will know that she is dying." With some hesitation I asked, "Bill, don't you think she knows?" He sighed deeply and said, "Please call him."

My call to Bill and Marie's parish was answered by a young clergyman who told me that he did not know Marie and Bill but that he would be right over. Briefly, I told him of their sense of separation from the church. While waiting for him to arrive, Bill and I returned to Marie's room. Doctors and nurses were moving actively around her, doing everything they could to comfort her in what they believed to be the final moments of her life.

"I'm here," Bill said, and then he moved to a chair near the foot of her bed. He didn't want her to know that he had been crying. Even now, he kept that distance, still believing he could protect her from the truth.

When their pastor arrived, he spent a few minutes alone with Marie and then asked us, along with some of the medical staff who were caring for Marie, to join them. As we gathered around Marie, we could sense her relaxing, even gaining strength as she struggled to participate. The priest asked each of us co-ministers to place our hands upon Marie. Placing the stole around his neck, he began the rites of the sacraments of the anointing of the sick and viaticum (Holy Communion for the dying).

As Marie received Holy Communion we listened to the petition, "May the body of Christ bring you to life everlasting." Marie's tears and smile washed over each one of us. Her reunion with Christ reconnected her to a source of peace and joy that she had known before. As each one of us gratefully accepted the final blessing, we knew we, too, had indeed been blessed.

The ordained minister then asked Marie and Bill to forgive the church for failing them in the past. The priest then said to Marie, "When you meet the Father, will you remember me? I'm finding it very hard to know his will; there is so much to be done." These beautiful petitions touched each of us deeply.

Marie did not die that day but lived for three more days. Bill never left her side; faithful in her dying as he had been faithful in her living. Now freed from his self-imposed isolation, he rubbed her back and repositioned her pain-filled body. He moistened her lips and stayed very close, sharing in the journey toward death. Bill also received a lot from Marie those final days. She listened, as he was now free to tell her the thoughts and feelings he had kept locked in his heart.

He told her of the rage he sometimes felt toward God and they prayed together for understanding and surrender. He tried to explain the confusion he felt regarding his anger toward her. He didn't blame her for her disease, and yet he found himself wanting to shout the words "How could you leave me? I need you and want you so." She understood. They talked, too, of those simple things of life — the practical concerns a wife has for her husband, his food and clothes; their home. "Take good care of yourself," she said.

They came together as a family once again. Their only child, a married son who had felt excluded during the long months of denial, was with them, expressing the powerful emotions repressed so painfully within him. At last it was okay to be honest and vulnerable with one another. The gift of trust belonged to them once more. Clearly, Marie finished the work of this life before she went, peacefully, to the Father. Assisted by the grace of the sacraments, she achieved reconciliation with the gifts of her life in relationship to God, her church, and her family.

Marie and Bill gave me a gift that has profoundly influenced and redirected my life. By allowing and accepting me into this sacred space in their lives, they enabled me to experience myself as minister. In the total ministry to this family I observed the beautiful blending between the personal and the sacramental, the lay and the ordained.

Though personal, the story of my call to, and preparation for, ministry to the sick contains common elements in the stories of other lay persons who are on a similar journey. The laity are coming to fuller participation in ministry in response to *the ordination of baptism*. We now have a deeper understanding of ministry. This is a result of our experience of being ministered to, and from knowing the emptiness of not having been ministered to, in our own pains. Most of us have come near, are in or beyond mid-life. No doubt this timing is linked to the psychological-spiritual tasks of this period in life. The search for meaning is often coupled with generativity, or the urge to care, not only for one's own, but for those beyond one's intimate family.

Lay Ministers: Something New or Very Old?

While on duty early one evening I came upon an elderly gentleman in our visiting clergy office. We have a register there so that lay ministers can record the names of the patients from their congregations that they have visited in order to link their visits with our staff chaplains. The gentleman, I observed, was writing in that register.

We introduced ourselves and he told me his name and the congregation he represented. I was aware that this congregation had recently begun a program for lay ministers who would visit the sick and so I responded, "Oh, yes, you must be one of the new lay ministers." "No," he replied quite emphatically, "I am not a minister, I am a member of the men's association. This is not new, I have been visiting the sick for twenty years. And," he continued quite emphatically, "I thought the pastors were ministers."

This encounter illustrates quite clearly that we are, once again, in a period of transition regarding the roles of the laity in the church. The transition includes a shift in language and language is vital for it defines our understanding. The gentleman from the men's association and I were not speaking the same language as we attempted to talk about similar issues. If he were to have described his role to me that evening he probably would have given an account something like this: he was bringing the concern of his congregation to those members he visits; he might offer to connect them or their family to the resources of their faith community for prayers, for healing, financial assistance, child care, or help in the home; he might share prayer during the visit and he may even be a good and significant listener. How then is his contact as a visitor any different from the visit of the lay minister from whom he so emphatically differentiates himself?

The differences, I believe, relate to the changes we are experiencing in the role and identity of the laity. When used in ecclesiastical language, the title "lay" is intended to connote nonordained status. This definition can be confused with another usage of the term "lay," meaning nonprofessional. For our purposes, "lay" will be used in the ecclesiastical sense, meaning nonclergy. In some ways the title "lay minister" is to the church as the term "high-tech" is to electronics. It is new. Ten years ago this language did not exist. The words *lay* and *minister* were mutually exclusive then. Today they are not.

Our English word *minister* comes from the Latin word *minister*, meaning "servant" or "helper." No reference to ordination is made. Current

usage of the word is further complicated by the denominational differences placed upon it. Protestants refer to their clergy as minister or pastor. Catholics refer to their clergy as priest or father. The Jews refer to
their clergy as rabbi (or teacher). Early in the Protestant tradition great
emphasis was placed upon the priesthood of all believers and yet the role
of priest has largely been borne by their clergy.

As we adapt to change we must redefine our words. Time, catechesis,
and the experience of the laity in ministry will be the levelers. We are
now calling and receiving lay persons to be the bearers of pastoral care
to the sick. Sounds like something new or is it the rebirth of something
very old?

Theologians continue to trace the changing roles of the laity and forms
of ministry within the church. In the early days of the church and continuing through the first millennium, the many and varied charisms of
the laity were identified, called forth, and utilized within the community. These ministries of service were performed in union with the ministries of the ordained. In his first letter to the Corinthians Paul defines
ministry not according to rank or status but *according to the individual
gifts we are given in the Spirit* (1 Cor 12:4-11). Each gift is a necessary
part, making up a whole body. Each and every gift must be respected,
cherished, and utilized in order to fulfill Christ's teachings.

By the second millennium the notion of actively representing Christ
to one another had shifted to the ordained men, and to the men and
women in religious orders. As their numbers increased, it appears that
the distinction was more easily made. The laity were to be ministered to,
the ordained were the ministers.

This surrendering of responsibility to exercise one's gifts in ministry
has been furthered in recent decades by the emergence of new categories of religious professionals: the ministries of the spiritual directors,
pastoral counselors, and hospital chaplains (many of whom are not ordained). The business of actively ministering to the crises, brokenness,
and suffering in our lives was best left to the skills and expertise of these
professionals. We might even speculate that the phrase, "I wanted to be
with my friend who was suffering but I was afraid I would say the wrong
thing," has resulted from this newborn professionalism. Having to say
the "right thing" emerges from the belief that professionals have been
educated to know the right thing to say.

Looking back over the history of the "care of souls," one is tempted to
see certain parallels in care of the body and the mind as well. During the
first millennium the laity assumed significant responsibility for their

own and others' physical wellbeing. Through the knowledge gained by oral tradition and trial and error, nonprofessionals ministered to the physical needs of one another (i.e., women assisted each other in pregnancy and childbirth; care of the physically and mentally impaired and of the aging and dying was a function of the family and the community). During the second millennium there is a significant shift in the care of the body. The development of medical science prepared physicians to be another class of experts. People were inclined to look to them to take full responsibility for physical well-being. In fact there seemed to be an attitude of indifference about one's body, not bothering to be attentive to physical needs. There was the expectation that when illness or accident struck, the physician would heal. Physicians and other health care professionals, the institutions they staff, gradually assumed responsibility for care of our bodies, just as the clergy assumed responsibility for our spiritual wellbeing.

The parallel can be drawn even further as we have seen the increased understanding and discoveries of psychological processes and the care of the mind. The availability of psychiatrists, psychologists — and other disciplines trained in counseling and mental health — has allowed us to look to yet another group of professionals to do much of what was once given freely among us. *The laity are moving to reclaim their responsibility in all three areas of caring, and are doing so quickly.* Though not new, lay ministry is countercultural. It challenges the professionalism of the day.

Lay Ministers at Lutheran General Hospital

Lay ministry at Lutheran General Hospital has undergone enormous growth and change in the past decade because the hospital is receptive to it and there are lay people ready and willing to accept the challenge. That ministry can be divided into three categories: parish visitors, auxiliary ministers of communion, full-time lay chaplains. Each is different, each has its own value.

Parish Visitors

Many parishes of all denominations have designated specific lay persons to visit hospitalized members of that parish. We continue to see their numbers multiply and to witness their faithfulness to their calling. This phenomenon is taking place in health care institutions across the country. Our hospital's Division of Pastoral Care has been adjusting and responding to their participation in ministry with us for several years. In order to facilitate their presence in our hospital as they visit members of their congregations, we offer some procedures and services.

An orientation meeting for lay ministers visiting on behalf of their congregation is offered annually to lay ministers from the forty congregations in the area. Our primary message in this meeting is to assure them of the value we place upon their ministry. This is demonstrated in several ways. They receive hospitality in our visiting clergy office and they are asked to use a register. The register is a tangible sign that we are interested in their ministry. It has a place for their name and phone number and the name of the congregation they represent. There is also a place for the name and room number of the members of their congregation whom they have visited. This method of accountability enables our chaplains to be in touch with the lay ministers from the parish, should the need arise, and is another statement of the importance placed upon their ministry.

Only those lay persons who have been authorized by their congregation may have access to our patient listings. They are required to wear a name tag that bears the name of their congregation, as well. Of course, the issues relating to patient rights and confidentiality are spelled out. In order that the lay ministers might be put at ease, they are given general guidelines for visiting in many specialized areas throughout the hospital (e.g., restrictions, identification of equipment, special garb to be worn, optimal times for visiting).

Probably the most valuable resource that is offered to these visiting lay ministers is the availability of a staff chaplain in the hospital twenty-four hours a day. They are encouraged to contact a chaplain immediately should they ever have serious concerns about a particular patient they have visited. This is extremely reassuring; it eases their anxieties about encountering a situation that they feel they cannot handle.

On occasion, either the hospital's pastoral care staff or the congregation may find it necessary to ferret out those individuals whose willingness exceeds their gifts to minister to the sick. This process may be painful, but necessary, if lay ministry is to continue to gain acceptance and credibility in the hospital. Such lay ministers are helped to identify other gifts that may be put to the service of their congregation.

Above all, we seek to reinforce the parish identity of the lay minister, to strengthen the link between that parish and the hospital. The walls that sometimes seem to isolate the patient from one's faith community can be significantly diminished by their ministries.

Auxiliary Ministers of Communion

In 1971 the Roman Catholic Church once again began to allow lay ministers to carry Holy Communion to the sick and to distribute Holy Communion at the mass. The utilization of the laity in this role is a vivid example of the blending of the new (personal) ministry with a very old (sacramental) ministry.

These ministers of care are called forth and endorsed by their parish priest and given approximately twelve hours of instruction on ministering to the sick. The ministers of care meet regularly in a group for peer support. The person leading the group may be a priest, sister, or lay person. Often this person has had Clinical Pastoral Education or related training, and is able to provide supervision.

The high visibility of these lay ministers (over two thousand in our Chicago area) who carry the sacrament from the liturgy to the sick has accelerated the entrance of lay persons from other denominations into ministry to the sick. Their ministry demonstrates and authenticates the need, the capability, and acceptability of lay persons doing the work that recent generations reserved for the ordained.

In addition to those auxiliary ministers of communion who carry communion from their own parish to their hospitalized parishioners is a second group whose ministry is to all hospitalized Catholic patients. Approximately thirty auxiliary ministers rotate the responsibility to provide communion to Catholic patients who are not being served by their own parish ministers. Their ministry is coordinated through the Division of Pastoral Care, but their primary identity and source of support is in their own parish. Our staff is, of course, available to them as needed. To acknowledge their work, Lutheran General Hospital invites them to a recognition dinner every year. In appreciation for their services they are also welcome to attend short courses offered by the Division of Pastoral Care, free of charge.

This group of lay ministers tends to be particularly faithful to their commitment. Their high degree of satisfaction in this ministry is, I believe, related to the clearly defined parameters of their work. They are responding to the patient's request to receive the sacrament, which gives them the benefit of being an invited, welcomed minister. The auxiliary ministers of communion do not seek to replace their parish clergy. Rather, they strive to maximize the caring resources of their congregation. Often they will mobilize their own pastor in particular situations.

Lay Chaplains

Lay ministers are serving in yet another capacity at Lutheran General Hospital: that of full-time lay chaplain.

This title was first used at our hospital in 1974 to identify the entry of lay persons into C.P.E. Lay ministers working in C.P.E. are peers of the clergy, religious, and seminary students in the program. They share in all of the functions of pastoral care. Since the word *chaplain* often presumes clergy status, the word *lay* is used to clarify the ecclesiastical status of the chaplain.

Lay ministers have continued to successfully complete C.P.E. programs (both quarter and one-year residency) the past nine years. Many of them have augmented their training with additional academic certification, particularly in the areas of theology and pastoral ministry. Several of these lay ministers have gone on to employment as lay chaplains in other hospitals, nursing homes, or parishes. A full-time lay chaplain is employed in the Division of Pastoral Care. Originally, the chaplain was to coordinate the ministry for Catholic patients. The need for such a particularly denominational ministry is the result of the traditional expectations of Catholic patients for a sacramental ministry while hospitalized. The lay chaplain coordinator utilizes the resources of the pastoral care staff, the local Catholic priests, and the lay ministers of care to facilitate this sacramental ministry and to blend it into the personal ministry of our staff chaplains.

Further, as the position was solidified, so its responsibilities were expanded to include ministry to families and staff of all faiths in the hospital's newborn intensive care unit. In this clinical responsibility, the lay chaplain functions as any other full-time staff chaplain assigned to other clinical areas.

Thirdly, this chaplain also has responsibilities for coordinating the training and supervision of all lay persons who provide ministry to the sick at Lutheran General Hospital.

Education for Lay Ministers

As lay ministries have grown, so have the needs for training and supervision. In response to this need Lutheran General Hospital's Division of Pastoral Care began a pilot training program in 1978: Clinical Ministry Education (C.M.E.). Its name suggests its relatedness to Clinical Pastoral Education which provides the structure for this program.

Clinical Ministry Education is a learning experience designed especially for lay persons who wish to enrich their personal ministry experiences through formal supervised training. C.M.E. functions on the basis of individually arranged educational contracts. Participant goals for each unit are stated in writing in order to begin negotiating these contracts. Personal goals are shared with the group during the first meeting. The broad program goals of C.M.E. are: (1) to understand the dimensions of ministry; (2) to reflect theologically about one's clinical experiences; (3) to develop the ability to more meaningfully communicate one's faith; (4) to explore and strengthen one's interpersonal relations; (5) to identify and evaluate one's assumptions about life; (6) to integrate clinical theory and practice.

The methodologies employed to attain these objectives include didactic sessions (led by lay and ordained staff chaplains), interpersonal growth groups (where feedback is provided on one's clinical work and group behavior), verbatim seminars (where written ministry interviews are discussed), case conference seminars (where situations of lay ministry are presented in more depth).

Participants in C.M.E. are granted graduate and undergraduate credit by several colleges in the area. Upon course completion, they also receive a certificate from the hospital. The course is offered in the fall and the spring and extends over a period of fourteen weeks, meeting once every week for three hours. In addition, each student is expected to spend approximately two hours each week in one's ministry (wherever that might be), which provides an important learning base for C.M.E.

The ecumenical spirit of C.M.E. has proven to be a rich, somewhat unexpected, resource for growth. Our denominational differences are of interest but do not in any way separate us. Our common efforts of ministry to the sick crystalize the elements that bind us together in our shared commitments to serve.

At mid-term written evaluations are shared. Each student evaluates his or her own experience and growth. These evaluation sessions tend to be most powerful. Clearly, they are impacted by the degree of trust that has been established in the group. The final evaluations, prepared and shared on the fourteenth week, tend to be somewhat anticlimactic. Participants have been sharing at various levels, openly and honestly with one another, and rarely save any surprises for this day. Final evaluations tend to be more transitional, as students are looking toward their future in ministry, with a vision expanded by this shared experience.

A few C.M.E. graduates have chosen to go on to take C.P.E. and further education to prepare for professional roles in lay ministries; however, the vast majority have returned to the parish/congregation to continue their original ministries, but with a new perspective and understanding.

Lay Ministry: The Challenge of the Third Millennium

As funding for hospital chaplaincy continues to shrink (see chap. 19 below), new and creative ways of utilizing lay ministries to the sick could be an obvious response. For instance, should we begin to call forth the gifts of ministry from our increasing population of older adults? It may be that a primary future role of ordained chaplains will be to mobilize, train, and enable lay persons to minister in our hospitals. By training and supervising teams of lay ministers, they will be able to maintain institutional ministry despite cutbacks in budgets and reduced numbers of full-time chaplains. There will be no reduction of patient needs in the future, no fewer people who will need to be touched. To meet such needs with reduced resources will call for creative and collaborative planning between churches and hospitals, between the ordained and the laity.

A Story of Ministry

Sarah, born three months earlier, had never left our newborn intensive care unit. Although she appeared to be a perfectly formed, beautiful infant, she suffered severe congenital anomalies that were incompatible with growth and life.

Although her parents had known, almost from the beginning, that she would never come home, they were not prepared for her sudden death before dawn one morning. Doctors and nurses had encouraged them to come into the hospital when they phoned them with the word of Sarah's death. The parents, overcome with shock and grief, had refused to come, saying that they chose to stay at home with their other daughters and to remember Sarah as she was when they had visited with her, the night before. However, when morning came they realized that they had to see her once more. I was notified when the parents arrived at the hospital while I was attending mass with a small group of staff patients and families in our chapel.

After brief and pain-filled moments of condolence and grief, I asked if they would want to stop in the chapel. Their refusal was swift, filled with confusion and rage. They asked then to be taken to see their dead baby. As we moved from the first-floor chapel area to the morgue in the basement, I remember noticing, as I had never done before, the contrast of these two sacred places. The main floor was carefully decorated with paintings, carpeting, plants—signs of life everywhere. As we approached the morgue, everything was so stark—bare walls and shining tile floors.

We found a small office for them and we talked a little in preparation for the unbelievable task that was ahead. After a while they indicated that they were ready. As I walked to the morgue I felt darkness, as if there would never be light, empty, almost without life myself.

The morgue attendant tenderly placed Sarah's body in a simple pink blanket and then into my arms. A wave of grief moved quickly over me. The harsh reality of death was enormous. As I moved across the hall, prayers of petition for Sarah's parents filled my heart. I paused at the door and found the parents clinging to one another, their faces filled with dread.

Soon I moved closer to them and bent over in order to bring the body of their infant near. As I uncovered her face the mother screamed out in her anguish, and, in response to her, I reached out and grasped her wrist tightly. As I did so, I suddenly realized that I was feeling her pulse and I was stunned by the sense of life and death, wholeness and brokenness that ensued. This heartbeat that had been life-giving for the child was now broken. The breath of life bursting forth in cries of agony from the mother; the breath of life now gone from the child. The body of the mother, so warm; the child so cold.

Just as it seemed that the suffering was more than could be endured, the experience was transformed in a gift of the Spirit to me. Suddenly I was reconnected beyond myself, back to our chapel where an ordained minister was celebrating the liturgy and remembering the mystery of our faith. God, our Father, gave Jesus, his Son, to life, suffering and death, so that we, like Sarah, might have life everlasting. *The stories of the past have meaning for the events of today.* The grace of this experience filled me with peace.

People and their needs do not vanish. They remain as stark realities of a life we hold in common. God's people are crying out to be touched by God's mercy. Lay people have no less responsibility or concern for the Maries, the Bills, the parents of the Sarahs of this world. Lay people want to join in the church's ministry to the oppressed and the anguished.

·PART IV·

THE HOSPITAL
CHAPLAIN
IN THE FUTURE

19

The Chaplain in the Future:
Threats and Opportunities

LAWRENCE E. HOLST

There will be fewer hospital chaplains around in the future. At least there will be fewer of them doing what they now do. This decline will not occur because of chaplains' incompetency or because of the public's disillusionment with their services. *The decline will have nothing to do with chaplains.* It will occur because there will be fewer hospitals, fewer occupied hospital beds, briefer hospitalizations, and reduced reimbursements for health care in the future. Most definitely, it will *not* be business as usual for the hospitals of the future. For that reason, it most definitely cannot be business as usual for the hospital chaplain of the future.

Human suffering will not decline. The numbers of sick people needing total health care will not diminish. But *who* delivers that care and *where* it is delivered will undergo marked changes for the remainder of this decade and on into the nineties. Being part of the establishment that delivers this care, hospital chaplaincy cannot, and should not, be immune to these changes.

Over the past twenty-five years, hospital chaplains have aligned themselves with the medical establishment. By and large, they sought and gained inclusion. As a result, most chaplains today find themselves on hospital, not church, payrolls. Though they retain connections with, and a loyalty toward, their own denomination, it has been an ecclesiastical, not a financial or administrative relationship.

The system has worked. Chaplains became much more accountable to hospitals; hospitals, in turn, became much more responsible for chaplaincy. Churches continued to educate and endorse clergy for specialized ministry, but hospitals hired them. Since their patients were receiving the services, patient revenues were used to pay chaplains. By being on hospital payrolls, chaplains qualified for wages and benefits that were generally attractive. The system worked, that is, so long as chaplains did their jobs to the satisfaction of administration and so long as patient revenues (usually through third-party reimbursements) were sufficient to cover such costs.

The "medical delivery revolution" that is now occurring has to do with third-party reimbursement. It is fast shrinking, as in turn will hospital services have to shrink. Chaplaincy is not being singled out as a target for declining reimbursements. However, by having chosen to be integrated into hospital budgets, chaplains and chaplaincy services cannot escape the impact. Shrinking reimbursements will accentuate internal competition for those reduced budgetary dollars. As a nonrevenue-producing department, chaplaincy will find itself at a distinct disadvantage.

The cause of this "reimbursement revolution" is money. Almost without exception the public feels that medical costs are too high. Hospitals are being singled out as the major culprit. It would appear that we have reached a point in America where hospitals are providing more health services than the public can (or chooses to) afford. We are in a curious period of expanding technology and shrinking resources. We are at a point where we can no longer equally balance *care, quality,* and *affordability.* The best we can do is to negotiate the most advantageous trade-offs between them.

In an effort to prod that negotiating process, third-party reimbursers (at this stage, Medicare) will limit their reimbursements. This, in turn, will compel hospitals to determine what services they can and will continue to provide. The new reimbursement methods will be prospective, commonly known as DRGs (diagnosis related groups). In each Medicare admission, a hospital will be told in advance what financial reimbursement it can expect to receive. To arrive at such a figure, all Medicare patients will be assigned to one of 467 newly defined diagnosis-related groups, based on the nature of their illness. Each DRG carries a specific rate of reimbursement. If the hospital can find a way to treat that patient for less, it can keep the profit. If the hospital's treatment costs more than the designated reimbursement, it must absorb the loss.

Reimbursement rates will be adjusted annually to reflect inflation and medical advances, as well as regional variations (to accommodate the higher costs of treatment in urban areas). As of this writing, psychiatric hospitals, long-term facilities, and rehabilitation centers are exempt from the new regulations. So are hospitals in Maryland, New York, and Massachusetts, which have their own cost containment programs in effect. A rather complex formula has been designed to change a patient's diagnostic group should medical complications arise. These, however, will be carefully monitored. To ease the adjustment for hospitals, prospective payments are being phased in over a three-year period. All hospitals are in the system as of 1 October 1984.

As of now, the new regulation applies only to Medicare patient admissions. However, since such admissions comprise about 40 percent of hospital revenues in our nation today, it already represents a significant impact. Furthermore, it is predicted that all third-party reimbursers (Blue Cross and commercial carriers) will follow suit and establish similar prospective payment systems.

If prospective payment is new, what has been the reimbursement system for hospitals in the past? It has been known as retrospective reimbursement. Under this system, the hospital determined its per diem costs (for labor, technology, equipment, space) and third-party carriers reimbursed at those rates. Audits of those costs were minimal. As might be expected, reimbursements varied from hospital to hospital, depending upon its own services and charges. There was little price competition between hospitals under retrospective payment. Third-party reimbursers paid the freight. Since out-of-pocket costs for the individual consumer (patient) were reduced or eliminated by insurance coverage, the patient demanded more and better services — regardless of costs — and hospitals sought to provide them. As might be expected, this system generated better services and higher costs. Today Americans spend $322 billion annually on health care, or an average of $1,200 per person. This represents 10.5 percent of America's gross national product.

How Did We Get This Way?

It has been suggested that any prognosis of the future must begin with a keen memory of the past, because the future grows out of the past. How did we get to this point where society is so adamant in its demands for hospitals to cut costs? How did hospitals get so out of touch with the public it is serving? Prior to World War II the community hospital was known as "the quiet place on the hill."[1] It was staffed with dedicated people, relatively underpaid, who fulfilled their responsibilities admirably and were held in high regard by the community. But those hospitals had no intensive care unit, no coronary care unit, no renal dialysis unit, no open heart surgery, no nuclear medicine, and not much of a laboratory. But there was, in most of them, much concern and comfort. There were also, in most of them, chronic financial problems. Their patients who could afford to paid more than the cost of the care they received, so that similar services could be provided to those who couldn't pay. It was involuntary, "Robin Hood philanthropy." Voluntary philanthropy and self-imposed taxes covered the balance of those hospitals' deficits.

More Hospitals

In 1946, with tax rates high but without the costs of a war, Congress looked for areas to direct those surplus revenues. One such area was hospital construction. The Hospital Survey and Construction Act (the Hill-Burton Bill) was passed. This was a huge subsidy program to encourage hospital construction. Scarcely a hospital was built in the fifties and sixties that did not receive a Hill-Burton grant and/or a low-interest government loan. Twelve billion dollars were spent on hospital construction from 1946 to 1973; 403,000 beds were added, doubling our nation's hospital bed capacity.[2]

More Services

It was not long before there was an acute need for people to staff these hospitals. The growth in medical services, and those trained to provide them, has been astonishing. Look around at any profession in the hospital today and trace its numerical growth over the past two decades and one will capture the incredible magnitude.

In 1960 there were approximately 250,000 active physicians; by 1980 there were 455,000, an increase of 82 per cent.

In 1970 there were 700,000 registered nurses; today there are about 1,339,000.

In 1965 there were 33,500 full-time therapists in hospitals; today there are over 251,000, an increase of 649 per cent.

In 1965 there were 88,900 clinical laboratory technologists; today there are about 276,000, a 210 per cent increase.

In 1965 there were 46,600 radiology technologists; in 1981 there were 104,000, a 123 per cent increase.

While no statistics were available for the 1960s, today there are over five thousand hospital chaplains in the United States.

As hospital beds grew, so did patient censuses, so did demands for services, so did the numbers of those trained to provide those services, so did costs.

More Technology

Not long afterward, Congress turned to scientific medical research. It was generous with its funds. Federal expenditures for health research expanded from $73 million in 1950 to $2 billion in 1972.[3] The funding has continued at that approximate level. These funds wrought a technological revolution in medical care. Indeed, technology was exploding in all sectors of life. Advances in one field spread to other fields. As a result of these advances, many hospitals today have intensive care units, with automatic electronic monitoring of all vital signs. They have renal dialysis units. They have artificial hearts, lungs, and kidneys. They have open heart surgery. They have radioisotopic scanning capabilities. They have laboratories that can perform two- to four-hundred different in vitro procedures, rapidly and accurately. An inestimable number of people are alive today who would not be were it not for these technological advances. But those advances did not come cheaply. Not only was capital funding needed to purchase equipment, but personnel were required to run the equipment. In 1950 hospitals employed less than two employees per patient bed; today that number has grown to four hospital employees per patient bed.[4]

More Entitlements

As more hospital beds, technology, and services were available, it became apparent to our government that many Americans did not have access to them—particularly the poor and the elderly. Congress again intervened. Title XVIII (Medicare) and Title XIX (Medicaid) were incorporated into the Social Security Act of 1965. These provided access to the rapidly growing medical services for the elderly and the poor. Every party had something at stake in these entitlements: the *patient* wanted the best care possible; the *hospitals* wanted to utlilize their vast technical and human resources; the *government* wanted equal access to these resources for all its citizens. But those stakes were expensive. In 1967 Medicare/Medicaid expenditures for health care were about $5 billion. By 1976 they were $33 billion. Today they are approximately $57.3 billion.

More Public Pressure

By the mid-1970s the climate and spirit had changed. Rather than expansion of medical services, there was a cry for retrenchment. Clearly, in the eyes of many, the entire health enterprise had gotten out of hand. Hospitals were singled out as major contributors to the spiraling costs. The then Secretary of Health, Education, and Welfare charged that "hospitals are obese," with an excess of 200,000 beds and with costs escalating at an annual rate of 14 percent. Hospitals found themselves in a crunch. The mood and the message had suddenly changed: encouraged by the Hill-Burton Act to construct more hospitals, they now found themselves overbedded; encouraged to develop technology and to expand services, they now found themselves costing the American public $322 billion annually; encouraged to make their medical services available to the elderly and the poor, they now faced a cap on Medicaid and Medicare reimbursements. Not only had the rules changed, the game changed. Little wonder that hospitals today have grown wary and weary. The pressures have been swift and sure.

Where Does That Leave Hospitals?

We have some broad hints as to what will happen to hospitals in the future.

They will be much more cost conscious:

Consumers will be encouraged by third-party reimbursers to shop for price. Industry estimates that $2,500 is spent per employee per year for health (including workmen's compensation). Employees will be given incentives to reduce those expenditures, which in turn, will impose price competition. Hospitals will need to increase their volume and decrease their per-patient costs, cutting costs to the bare bone, without compromising quality. As one leader in the field put it: "Hospitals will be lean and mean."

They will be more competitive and entrepreneurial:

Hospitals will be in competition for patients, and they will seek to broaden their economic base by acquiring companies and marketing products/services that can turn a profit.

They will be narrower in scope of medical services:

Each hospital will determine what it can do best and most efficiently and do it. It will be increasingly difficult to be medically heterogeneous in scope and survive.

They will be fewer in number:

It is predicted that one in seven hospitals will be out of business by 1990. Those that survive will become a part of massive coalitions and networks, making it difficult for the local hospital to retain its unique identity and mission.

They will care for fewer in-patients for briefer periods of time:

Some predict that in-patient admissions will be cut by one third. It is estimated that 30 percent of today's hospitalized patients do not really need to be there; certainly that group will not be there tomorrow. Nationally the average length of stay has already reduced from 9.2 days in 1972 to a current 8.3 days. Further reductions are anticipated.

They will be physically focused:

George Caldwell, President of Lutheran General Health Care Systems, sees the danger of tomorrow's hospital becoming "a body shop." There will be no reward for doing a more humane job or for addressing quality-of-life issues. Payment will come for healing the body. Health care will be narrowly defined. The thrust will be on profit, efficiency, and standardization.

They will house the acutely ill who only can be treated there:

A smaller portion of health care will be delivered in the hospital. More services will be offered by hospitals outside the hospital. Surgical patients will come in the day of surgery. Many will go home the same day. Diagnostic work-ups, tests, X rays, lab work will be done prior to admission.

They will take services into the home:

To expedite early discharge, hospitals will need to provide follow-up home care, including physician and nurse house calls for treatment. Families will be assisted to provide part of the convalescent care.

The hospital of tomorrow will be tested as never before. It will confront the contradictory demands of the public for "high tech" and "high touch" at low costs. Clearly, services, and perhaps quality, will be lowered. Admittedly, it is a grim picture. Admittedly, it is a speculative picture. Admittedly, public moods and temperaments can and do shift, as do national priorities. But it is clear today that the public is opting for lower medical costs. To miss that is to be naive. How much that will impact quality and comprehensiveness of care, no one knows. And if that impact is severe — as many predict — who knows what the public's next mandate will be?

Where Does That Leave Chaplains?

Certainly, this leaves hospital chaplains with more questions than answers. To be sure, there will always be hospitals and people who need to be in them. Likewise, there will always be a need for chaplains to bring comfort and care to such people. *Hospital chaplaincy is not going out of business. But it will indeed change.* In all likelihood, there will not be as many chaplains doing tomorrow what they've been doing in the past. Hospital budgets simply won't allow it. This will be particularly true for those hospitals that have large pastoral care staffs. This will even be true for those chaplaincy programs that are financially underwritten, totally or partially, by the church. For as programs formerly underwritten by hospitals are cut or reduced, more will turn to synods and denominations for funding. Chaplaincy in the future will need to broaden two bases: *clinical* and *financial.* Like any change, corporate or individual, this will pose threats and opportunities.

Broaden the Clinical Base

As hospitals need to broaden their base of services, so will the chaplain. Chaplains can be no less creative than hospitals. If fewer people are going to spend fewer days in tomorrow's hospital (and there is no anticipated cutback in illness), then people are going to be treated somewhere. The chaplain will need to pursue that somewhere.

That somewhere will be out-patient facilities. Considerable diagnostic and treatment work will be done upon patients who "commute." These will include surgeries, workups, testings, and therapies. These will occur in soon-to-be-expanded out-patient facilities. In sharp contrast to the past, there will be disincentives to hospitalize such patients. Yet these patients, and their families, will face the same anxieties and have the same needs that in-patients have today who go through the same procedures. In the future these patients will be a less captive audience. The chaplain will have to go looking for them. Instead of bedsides, chaplains will minister in lobbies, waiting rooms, and small but active treatment areas.

The patient needs will not change, only the context. The chaplain will need to develop entries into the context. But hospital chaplains are not unprepared for such a context, for they have considerable experience in taking initiative and providing ministry in unstructured, informal ways. Chaplains have expertise in effecting significant encounters within minutes. That will prove to be helpful, for often minutes are all they will have with such patients.

That somewhere will also be the home. Earlier discharges (mandated by prospective payment) will transfer more care to the home. Home care departments, formerly ancillary, will become focal. Hospitals will organize health care teams that will continue *treatment* into the patient's home. That means doctors, nurses, and therapists of many kinds making house calls on a routine basis. Not at all will this be disadvantageous to patients. But it will mean considerable adjusting for health care personnel who will lose many of the conveniences of the hospital. It will be an adjustment, as well, for the families who, in the past, have delegated such caring responsibilities to the hospital.

It will provide an excellent opportunity for pastoral care. The warm, stabilizing support of a sensitive chaplain, visiting regularly in the home, may make the difference in enlarging the capacities of those families to cope. Most chaplains come out of the parish ministry where home visits are routine. They may now become routine again. Indeed, it is just possible that chaplains will feel more at home in the home than they feel in hospitals.

Chaplains also have training and experience as facilitators of care. Families, parishioners, and community resources will need to be mobilized and trained to care for such patients. Chaplains could be links to such care, and such care will be needed.

It is ironic that financial exigencies will cause history to repeat itself. At the turn of this century only those without family support were hospitalized, the others were sent home to the care of their families. Hospitals were for the poor. For obviously different reasons today, much convalescent medical care will return to the home. The chaplain has an important role on such ambulatory health teams. But that role needs to be identified. I would see it as providing direct care and facilitating the care of others. A new supportive role awaits parishes for families of the suffering. Hospital chaplains can help identify that need and train parishioners to fill it.

That somewhere will be with employees. Most hospitals have employee assistant programs (E.A.P.). These have been organized both for altruistic and ulterior motives. They are ways of caring, but they also help to keep employees healthy and on the job. It has been found that early detection and intervention can often prevent employees' personal problems from escalating. Such problems may be home or work related, intrapsychic, interpersonal, familial, or financial. Whatever the source of the problem, its effects are bound to spread, eroding work efficiency. So hospitals, and other corporations, have learned that it is in their self-interest to keep employees well, to help them effectively cope with stresses and crises in their lives. Over the years chaplains have provided care and counseling to hospital employees, often informally. The time has come for the pastoral function to be formalized. Chaplains are valuable resources in employee assistance programs. Many have the administrative ability to manage them. Such programs continue to provide important areas for pastoral care in hospitals.

In addition, chaplains will need to be available, as in the past, to help staff with stress points in patient care. It has always been difficult to be surrounded by needy people. It will be even more so in the future when hospital personnel will be called upon to do more in less time and with fewer resources.

That somewhere will be the field of medical ethics. Hospitals will face enormous ethical issues in the future. External forces will compel hospitals to formalize multidisciplinary bioethics committees, whose power and influence will grow. Such committees will, in all likelihood, include community representation. Because such issues involve legal, moral, religious, financial, and medical factors, it is rare that any single person is equipped and informed in all those related fields. Yet someone needs to assert leadership. In many hospitals chaplains are the most qualified persons to chair such committees. Their combined theological, moral, and philosophic background, coupled with their clinical experience, renders many of them sufficiently competent to meet such a demanding task. It will not be easy. A theological degree does not turn one into a medical ethicist. Issues will need to be researched, position papers will need to be written, seminars will need to be held, links to the day-to-day clinical world will need to be maintained, homework will need to be done. These will be demanding and time consuming. The point is not that it will be easy, but that chaplains are persons who can help hospitals meet such complex bioethical issues.

That somewhere will be in administration. Though their formal training in administration is not extensive, most chaplains have a keen sensitivity for many administrative functions, i.e., interpersonal relations, group process, defining and evaluating goals, organizing and motivating people around prescribed tasks. Many of them already hold administrative responsibilities beyond their own departments. Some chair multidisciplinary committees, others are clinical coordinators; some have responsibilities for long-range planning, others help write hospital policies; some serve as links to the wider community, others are on grievance committees. Chaplains provide hospitals with a reservoir of administrative/organizational talent that may need to be more visible and made more available in the future.

That somewhere will be with the elderly. In the next fifty years the general population in the United States is expected to grow by 35 percent, the over-age sixty-five by 119 percent and the over-age eighty-five by 206 percent. By the year 2,000 life expectancy is predicted to reach 72.9 for males (as compared to 69.5 today) and 81.1 for females (as compared to 77.2 today). This aging population wants, and will continue to want, to stay in their homes as long as possible rather than to be permanently institutionalized. This means that hospital utilization by the elderly will increase. Periodic hospitalization will better enable them to maintain independent living arrangements. Already one third of the nation's health care expenditures and one half of the federal health care expenditures are committed to those over age 65. Per capita hospital expenditures for the elderly are over three and a half times higher than for patients under 65. Hospital admission rates are three times higher for the elderly and their average length of hospital stay is five days longer.

The trend has already developed; it will continue. Chaplains will need to learn more about this sector of our population, for they will continue to comprise the majority of our hospitalized patients. This must include intergenerational ministry and follow-up care. Choice of hospital may be made, in part, on the quantity and quality of spiritual care provided this influential age group.

That somewhere will be in hospital image-building. The hospital of the future will need to act and be more businesslike. The margin for financial miscalculation will grow smaller. Such pressures are bound to impact the attitudes and outlooks of those who work in hospitals. Yet hospitals will remain service organizations. Their major product will continue to be personalized care. To help call attention to that primary focus in the midst of cutbacks will be a primary task of the chaplain. To help see to it that services are humanized, that a bureaucracy is personalized, that a caring image is projected in the community, will be a much needed function of pastoral care in a hospital. It will be needed by our health care delivery system as never before. To find ways to do this, individually and corporately, will be the most demanding challenge facing the chaplain tomorrow.

Broaden the Financial Base

It may be necessary in the future for chaplains to become direct revenue producers. Certainly, this will appear threatening to the vast majority of hospital chaplains whose budgets in the past have been provided by others' revenue production. What skills can a chaplain market, and to whom? That will be a crucial question tomorrow. The answer can only come by an analysis of one's own skills and of the needs of the community.

An obvious market is the parish. Chaplains may need to partially subsidize their salaries through services rendered to parishes. These services could include counseling (individual, marriage, family), crisis intervention, education (conducting seminars on stress management, family relationships, value clarification, wellness, personality development), intrastaff relations, and lay training. Such services could be rendered to individual parishes or to clusters of parishes. As with most things mentioned in this chapter, chaplains have often served in the past as consultants to parishes as time permitted. It was more by choice than necessity. Such a ministry may now need to be carefully formalized and marketed. It may become a necessity.

The chaplain of tomorrow may have to raise funds for chaplaincy. That is an awesome and gruesome prospect, but a realistic one. Sources of funding will vary: local parishes, foundations, individuals, corporations. Where chaplaincy has made a significant impact in a community over time, such a task may not be so awesome as anticipated. Many chaplaincy departments today are seeking to underwrite various programs through endowments. We need to make those efforts known to one another. We need to benefit from one another's experience.

Finally, in this regard, a blunt word needs to be spoken to the national and local church. During the growth of the past three decades hospitals have paid the freight for chaplaincy and Clinical Pastoral Education. Or, to be more accurate, the public has paid the freight. This has been an involuntary contribution. Patients have not consented to it. Most of them probably did not even know that a portion of their hospital bill went toward chaplaincy and pastoral education. In all of this the church has been a hitchhiker. Today, thousands of pastors, of all denominations, serving in institutions and parishes, have received clincial training in hospitals at the public's expense. Those sources of public reimbursement are shrinking. What is to be the role of the church?

In those growth decades churches and chaplains have coexisted, but with little dynamic interaction. It was a luxury that both could afford. That luxury can no longer be afforded. The day of separatism is over. The church will need to invest more of its energies and funds in chaplaincy and Clinical Pastoral Education; chaplains will need to identify more closely with the church. But that, too, provides opportunities for mutual enrichment. Each needs the other: the church needs institutional chaplaincy to reach a segment of society untouched by the parish; the chaplain needs the church for theological mooring and mission renewal, as well as personal (and maybe financial) support.

Healing has always been a vital mission of the church. That is well demonstrated by the fact that the church has established more hospitals than any other agency on earth. Chaplaincy has been, and will continue to be, a vital link to that vital mission of the church.

Surely, what appears above does not exhaust the frontiers awaiting chaplains in the future. There are many more. Nor is there intended a suggestion that any one chaplain or chaplaincy department move into all of these frontiers. Each of us must be creatively selective. Nor am I suggesting that traditional in-patient ministry be abandoned. After all, such ministry, effectively done, has largely accounted for the affirmation chaplaincy has received within the hospital. As John Gleason, Jr., points out: "Nothing makes a believer of an administrator, physician, nurse or paitent than first-hand experience of tangible services (i.e., the calming of an upset patient or improving the attitude of a troubled employee)."[5]

What seems apparent is that hospital chaplains, as never before, will need to prioritize and deploy scarcer resources to meet changing and expanding needs. That's tomorrow's threat and opportunity.

Conclusion

There are two dangers in writing such a chapter: it may appear to invalidate the rest of the book; and, its predictions may turn out to be wrong. Of the second danger little can be said. Predictions can only be those and nothing more. Currents and trends may change as quickly in the last half of this decade as they did in its first half. Only time will tell.

However, in no way, do these predictions invalidate concepts and practices carefully depicted in this book. There is no doubt in my mind that hospital chaplaincy will continue in the near and distant future for at least two reasons: (1) there will continue to be needs for it — suffering will not be abated in the future; and (2) it has demonstrated in the past a capacity to meet many such needs.

There is also no doubt in my mind that hospital chaplaincy will need to be modified. That will be necessary because the context in which it is offered is being modified. In many ways, hospital chaplains face a crisis not dissimilar to the patients to whom they minister. Change and threats abound. The demands to adapt and grow are compelling. Like patients, chaplains will face new boundaries and limits. They, too, will need to make peace between their infinite aspirations and their finite possibilities. Like patients, chaplains have resources. Through their daily experiences with life and death, suffering and loss, chaplains have learned to cope with change. Like patients, chaplains must contend with a changing self-image. Over the years, chaplains have struggled long and hard with self-doubts and with the doubts of others about their legitimacy in health care. The struggle was fought and won. The chaplain's place and role in the hospital has won broad acceptance. But that place has changed. Now chaplains face new struggles, new limits, and new challenges. Like the patients to whom they minister, chaplains face ominous threats to the old patterns and enormous opportunities for new life and growth. Like so many patients, chaplains need new visions and the will to pursue them.

NOTES

1. "The Decline and Demise of the Community Hospital," *Insights* by J. Lloyd Johnson Associates, 1978, p. 1.

2. Ibid. p. 2.

3. Ibid. p. 2.

4. *Health in the United States*, Health Resources Administration, D. H. E. W. 76-1232, Washington, D. C., 1976, p. 2.

5. John J. Gleason, Jr., "The Marketing of Pastoral Care, Counseling, Chaplaincy and C.P.E.," *Journal of Pastoral Care* 38, no. 4 (1984): 265.

DATE DUE